AF870834

Pericarditis - Diagnosis and Management Challenges

Edited by Alexander E. Berezin

Published in London, United Kingdom

Pericarditis - Diagnosis and Management Challenges
http://dx.doi.org/10.5772/intechopen.104157
Edited by Alexander E. Berezin

Contributors
Erhan Hafiz, Ozgur Altinbas, Michael R. Sood, Daniel Zinkovsky, Siddharth Pahwa, Juliana Cobb, Francesco Maria Lauri, Onur Benli, Mouna Snoussi, Yosra Bouattour, Zouhir Bahloul, Andrew O. Maree, Jack Hartnett, Richard Armstrong, Lisa Brandon, Igor F. Palacios, Hani Jneid, Christopher J. Palestro

© The Editor(s) and the Author(s) 2023

The rights of the editor(s) and the author(s) have been asserted in accordance with the Copyright, Designs and Patents Act 1988. All rights to the book as a whole are reserved by INTECHOPEN LIMITED. The book as a whole (compilation) cannot be reproduced, distributed or used for commercial or non-commercial purposes without INTECHOPEN LIMITED's written permission. Enquiries concerning the use of the book should be directed to INTECHOPEN LIMITED rights and permissions department (permissions@intechopen.com).

Violations are liable to prosecution under the governing Copyright Law.

(cc) BY

Individual chapters of this publication are distributed under the terms of the Creative Commons Attribution 3.0 Unported License which permits commercial use, distribution and reproduction of the individual chapters, provided the original author(s) and source publication are appropriately acknowledged. If so indicated, certain images may not be included under the Creative Commons license. In such cases users will need to obtain permission from the license holder to reproduce the material. More details and guidelines concerning content reuse and adaptation can be found at http://www.intechopen.com/copyright-policy.html.

Notice

Statements and opinions expressed in the chapters are these of the individual contributors and not necessarily those of the editors or publisher. No responsibility is accepted for the accuracy of information contained in the published chapters. The publisher assumes no responsibility for any damage or injury to persons or property arising out of the use of any materials, instructions, methods or ideas contained in the book.

First published in London, United Kingdom, 2023 by IntechOpen
IntechOpen is the global imprint of INTECHOPEN LIMITED, registered in England and Wales, registration number: 11086078, 5 Princes Gate Court, London, SW7 2QJ, United Kingdom

British Library Cataloguing-in-Publication Data
A catalogue record for this book is available from the British Library

Additional hard and PDF copies can be obtained from orders@intechopen.com

Pericarditis - Diagnosis and Management Challenges
Edited by Alexander E. Berezin
p. cm.
Print ISBN 978-1-83768-363-5
Online ISBN 978-1-83768-364-2
eBook (PDF) ISBN 978-1-83768-365-9

We are IntechOpen, the world's leading publisher of Open Access books

Built by scientists, for scientists

6,400+
Open access books available

173,000+
International authors and editors

190M+
Downloads

156
Countries delivered to

Our authors are among the
Top 1%
most cited scientists

12.2%
Contributors from top 500 universities

CLARIVATE ANALYTICS
BOOK CITATION INDEX
INDEXED

WEB OF SCIENCE™

Selection of our books indexed in the Book Citation Index
in Web of Science™ Core Collection (BKCI)

Interested in publishing with us?
Contact book.department@intechopen.com

Numbers displayed above are based on latest data collected.
For more information visit www.intechopen.com

Meet the editor

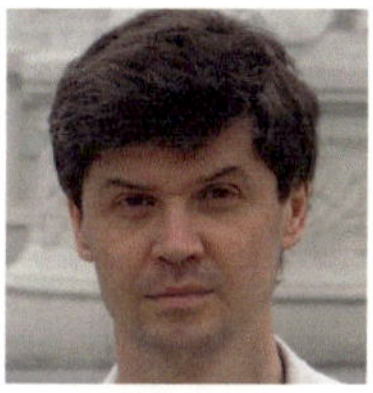

Alexander E. Berezin received his MD degree in 1992, and his DSci specializing in heart failure in 2004, both from State Medical University, Zaporozhye, Ukraine. He is a Professor of Medicine and Senior Consultant in the Internal Medicine Department at Zaporozhye State Medical University. He is a fellow of the ESC, the Ukrainian Cardiology Association, and a member of its working group on atherosclerosis and vascular biology. His research interests include the fundamental study of heart failure and biomarkers. He is the current editor-in-chief of *Biological Markers and Guided Therapy, Diabetes Research and Treatment*, and a board member for *World Journal of Diabetes, World Journal of Cardiology* and other highly reputed international medical journals.

Contents

Preface

Pericarditis, the commonest form of pericardial disease with known infectious or noninfectious causes, and an idiopathic etiology, is on the rise across the world. Although the approaches to diagnosis and management of acute and chronic pericarditis are well established and reported in international clinical guidelines, there is a large number of unresolved issues in these fields. For instance, clinical criteria, including signs and symptoms, the presence of specific physical findings such as pericardial rub, electrocardiographic changes and echocardiographic evidence for hemodynamic modality and pericardial effusion or constriction, do not specifically correspond to the etiology and natural evolution of the disease. Yet, the etiology of some idiopathic cases may be defined as viral, including COVID-19, and may also be associated with long Covid, tuberculosis, neoplasm, systemic vasculitis and connective tissue diseases. In fact, variable diagnostic tests seem to be highly specific and sensitive if no specific etiologies are suspected in connection with the epidemiological background, patient history and clinical presentation. This book presents a summary of conventional diagnostic and treatment approaches in acute, chronic and recurrent pericarditis, with a particular focus on clinical practice utilization.

Alexander E. Berezin
Professor of Medicine and Senior Consultant,
Internal Medicine Department,
Zaporozhye State Medical University,
Zaporozhye, Ukraine

Section 1

Etiologic Diagnosis and Practical Aspects of the Management of Acute Pericarditis

Chapter 1

Acute Pericarditis

Erhan Hafiz and Ozgur Altinbas

Abstract

Pericardium is a double-layered anatomic structure that surrounds the heart and output sections of the great vessels. Despite numerous functions of this layer, mains are the protection of the heart and facilitation of the heart movements. Various diseases were defined related to the pericardium and one of them is acute pericarditis caused by inflammation of the pericardium mostly by infection. In this chapter, it is aimed to give brief information about the mostly seen pericardial diseases and detailed information about the signs, symptoms, diagnosis, and treatment modalities about the acute pericarditis.

Keywords: pericardium, acute pericarditis, infection, inflammation, effusion

1. Introduction

Pericardium is a flask-shaped structure that contains the heart and the proximal parts of the great vessels. Various functions of the pericardium were defined such as stabilization of the heart in its correct anatomic position by maintaining the suitable geometry of the heart and providing the pressure-volume correlation of the cardiac chambers. It also acts as a barrier to protect the heart from spread of infections and neoplasms born of mediastinum. It prevents the abrasion of the surface of the heart due to the movements of the heart by the fluid in pericardial cavity. This fluid contains prostoglandines which is secreted by endothelial and mesothelial cells of the pericardium and regulates the cardiac reflexes, contractile function of the myocardium, and coronary tone of the epicardium [1–3].

Various systemic and cardiac disorders can affect the pericardium. Occasionally, pericardium itself can be locus of isolated disease. Pericardial responses to the detrimental agent are usually acute pericardial inflammation called pericarditis or pericardial effusion whereas both of them often occur together. In addition, if a response of acute pericardial inflammation does not regress, a chronic process includes microscopic fibroproliferation followed by macroscopic thickening can take place [4].

Acute inflammation of the pericardium, namely acute pericarditis may occur with or without pericardial effusion. It may manifest a systemic disease or an isolated clinical issue. Although multiple causes were defined in the literature underlying factors of acute pericarditis, 90% of the cases are virally originated or idiopathic. Correct and rapid diagnosis may help to prevent undesirable conditions such as recurrent pericarditis and pericardial construction [5].

Acute pericarditis is diagnosed in nearly 0.1% of hospital admissions and 5% of the patients admitted to emergency department with noncardiac chest pain. Bacterial causes are rarely detected in the pericarditis cases in developed countries, however especially tuberculosis is widely found to be the cause of the disease in developing countries. Mortality rate of the acute pericarditis for in-hospital patients was found to be 1.1% [6–8].

The purpose of this chapter is to give brief data about the anatomy, histology, and diseases related to pericardium and then broad description about acute pericarditis by reviewing the literature.

2. Anatomy and the histology of the pericardium

The pericardium is a double-layered structure which surrounds the heart and the roots of great vessels. Outer layer consists of connective tissue and called fibrous pericardium and the inner layer consists of serous membrane and called serous pericardium. Serous pericardium has two layers; parietal and visceral layers. Pericardial fluid takes part between these layers [9]. Pericardium itself and its fluid protect the heart against trauma, infection, maintain the stable position of the heart in the mediastinum, and provide lubrication for heart movements [10].

The pericardium also prevents the both overfilling of the heart which can be resulted in low cardiac output and excessive heart dilatation [11]. The pericardiophrenic artery is the main artery of the pericardium and its venous drainage goes into the azygos and internal thoracic veins. Phrenic nerve innervates the pericardium [12].

The amount of the pericardial fluid in adult humans is approximately between 20 and 60 mL (average 15–35 mL) and transudate in nature. Over the half of the cells involved in pericardial fluid are lymphocytes and others are granulocytes, macrophages, eosinophils, basophils, and mesothelial cells [13].

Anterior parietal pericardium is composed of three layers; serosa, fibrosa, and epipericardial connective tissue layer. The serosa includes a surface layer of mesothelial cells, the fibrosa contains collagen and small elastic fibers, and the epicardial connective tissue consists of large bundles of collagen that is the part of pericardiocostal ligament. Electron microscopic examinations showed that mesothelial pericardial cells have unique cilia and covered with microvilli which increases the surface area for transportation of fluid and assumes friction [14]. Mesothelial monolayer generates the visceral pericardium which adheres firmly to the epicardium. Mesothelial cells present in the pericardium are metabolically active and play role in myocardial contractility and modulation of symphatetic neurotransmission by producing endothelin, prostacyclin, eicosanoids, and prostaglandin E_2 [15].

3. Diseases of the pericardium

Pericardial diseases can be categorized as acute pericarditis, pericardial effusion, constrictive pericarditis, and cardiac tamponade. Afterward recurrent or chronic pericarditis can be developed in patients. Congenital structural pericardial abnormalities and pericardial cysts are occasionally seen and usually symptom-free [16].

3.1 Congenital structural defects of the pericardium

Congenital defects of the pericardium are uncommon conditions and classified as the size and the location of the defect such as complete or partial absence of the pericardium and right or left-sided pericardium. This condition does not change the life expectancy, however in particular cases strangulation and herniation of the cardiac chambers can cause life-threatening situations like sudden cardiac death [17].

Treatment differs from patient's signs and symptoms, and the location and the size of the defect [18].

3.2 Pericardial cysts

Cysts of the pericardium are rarely seen congenital masses located in the mediastinum.

Although it is usually asymptomatic it may have severe complications like obstruction of the main bronchi and right ventricle outflow tract, tamponade, and abrupt cardiac death due to size and the location of the lesion. Treatment approaches include follow-up if the patient is asymptomatic and drainage and/or resection if becomes symptomatic [19].

3.3 Pericardial tamponade

Pericardial tamponade is a clinical situation where the intrapericardial fluid accumulation raises the pressure surrounding the heart and compromises cardiac filling. Markedly elevated venous pressures result by compression of the heart cause impaired cardiac output producing cardiogenic shock which can be fatal [5]. The most common causes of the pericardial tamponade are malignancies, idiopathic pericarditis, and uremia [20]. The amount of the fluid that causes the pericardial tamponade differs 100–1000 cc according to the thickening and the stretching features of the pericardium. It may occur with less amount of fluid in patients with recurrent pericarditis due to scar formation [21].

Beck's triad aids in the diagnosis of the cardiac tamponade; decrease in the systemic blood pressure, increase in the systemic venous pressure and diminished heart sounds [22]. However, echocardiography is the gold standard of diagnosis [23].

Treatment of the pericardial tamponade upon the removal of the fluid. This can be performed either by pericardiocentesis or sub-xiphoidal surgery. Resuscitative thoracotomy can be used in emergency department to whom with traumatic arrest [24].

3.4 Pericardial effusion

Pericardial effusion is the accumulation of fluid in the pericardial sac more than it should. Although variety of etiologic factors were defined in the literature lead to pericardial effusion such as infection, inflammation, neoplasms, trauma, cardiac and vascular disorders, many cases of pericardial effusion are idiopathic [25]. Beside, pericardial effusion due to tuberculosis is more common in developing countries while postoperative complications and viral infections that cause pericardial effusion are prevalent in developed countries [26]. Because of the limited elasticity, in acute settings, lesser amount of fluid (100–150 mL) can cause cardiac tamponade. In chronic situations when the accumulation is gradual, the parietal pericardium has enough time to stretch, so pericardial effusion may become over 1 L before it causes tamponade [27]. Tachycardia, increased jugular venous pressure, pulsus paradoxus, orthopnea, and pericardial rub (only in pericarditis) are the main signs and symptoms of the pericardial effusion. Bradycardia and hypotension are usually seen before cardiac arrest [28].

Primary diagnostic tool for pericardial diseases including pericardial effusion remains echocardiography because of its portability, availability, and limited costs. In addition, computed tomography and cardiac magnetic resonance imaging allow the detection of loculated effusion, pericardial masses, and thickening and associated chest abnormalities by providing larger field of view [25].

Treatment approaches to the pericardial effusion based on underlying disease if it is detectable. If the diagnosis is idiopathic or unclear with elevated inflammatory markers aspirin or non-steroidal anti-inflammatory drugs can be initial therapy which also allows evaluating the response. In the circumstance of recurrent inflammatory situation initial therapy is recommended to be aspirin or non-steroidal anti-inflammatory drugs with colchicine. If accompying status such as pregnancy or systemic inflammatory disease, corticosteroids at low to moderate doses can be added. Corticosteroids are also be used if there is intolerance or contraindication to aspirin or non-steroidal anti-inflammatory drugs or failure with those drugs. Methotrexate and azathioprine are the other treatment choices [29–32].

3.5 Constrictive pericarditis

Constrictive pericarditis is characterized by fibrosis, scarring, calcification, and loss of elasticity of pericardium which leads to external impedance of heart that inhibits diastolic filling [33]. In the past, tuberculosis played an important role in the etiology of constrictive pericarditis, however today other causes such as thoracic irradiation and previous open heart surgeries are other common causes of the disease. But most cases still seemed to be idiopathic in origin [34].

Various clinical manifestations are related to constrictive pericarditis. These may be associated with volume overload that leads to weight gain or sweating or in association with decreased cardiac output that leads to dyspnea on exertion and fatigue. In addition, congestive hepatomegaly and/or ascites may cause abdominal discomfort. Peripheral edema may also be present. Echocardiography is the best-recommended test for the diagnosis of constrictive pericarditis as in any other pericardial diseases [35].

Exact management of chronic constrictive pericarditis is pericardiectomy with removing as much of pericardium as possible. Myocardial penetration with calcification and fibrosis are the worse prognostic factors. Diuretics can be used to decrease edema. Besides, anti-inflammatory treatment up to 3 months with close follow-up should be started a hemodynamically stable patient with newly diagnosed constrictive pericarditis [36].

4. Acute pericarditis

In general, inflammation of the pericardial sac described as pericarditis. It is the most common pathologic course involving the pericardium. If the duration of pericarditis lasts for less than 4–6 weeks, it is called “acute pericarditis”. Subacute pericarditis is the disease in which the pericarditis lasts for more than 4–6 weeks but less than 3 months. Chronic pericarditis continues more than 3 months. If there is an asymptomatic intervals of 4–6 weeks between episodes then the term “recurrent pericarditis” is used [18].

4.1 Etiology

According to the 2015 European Society of Cardiology guidelines, etiology of the acute pericarditis was divided into two fundamental groups; infectious and non-infectious causes. Viral infections are the most common cause of the acute infectious pericarditis. Various types of viral agents were defined that lead to acute pericarditis such as coxsackie A and B viruses, adenoviruses, echoviruses, parvovirus B19, influenza viruses, human immunodeficiency virus, cytomegalovirus, and Ebstein-Barr virus [37]. Bacterial microorganisms lead to pericarditis are rarely seen in developed countries however tuberculosis is still considered to be the most common cause of pericarditis in the endemic part of the developing countries. Beside, pneumococcus, *Coxiella burnetii*, meningococcus, streptococcus, and staphylococcus are the other bacterial causes of pericarditis which can appear as purulent tamponade with life-threatening clinical situations [38]. Fungal and parasitic organisms rarely cause acute pericarditis. Histoplasma, Candida, Coccidioides, Blastomyces, Toxoplasmosis, and Echinococcus species can be given as examples of causative agents [39].

Various non-infectious factors that lead to acute pericarditis were described in the literature. The mains are malignancy especially secondary to metastasis, connective tissue disease, and metabolic causes [6].

Blunt-force trauma is supposed to be another cause of acute pericarditis. The clinic becomes apparent days or weeks after initial injury. Pathophysiology of the post-traumatic pericarditis is thought to be autoimmune but exact mechanism still remains unclear [40].

Dressler syndrome is a form of acute pericarditis which happens as a result of injury to pericardium or heart following cardiac surgery or myocardial infarction. It is also called post-myocardial infarction syndrome with delayed inflammatory response usually present greater than 2 weeks after the initial event [41].

Several medications were defined as cause to drug-induced pericarditis. Drugs such as hydralazine, isoniazid, and procainamide cause to lupus-like syndrome which is associated with pericardial involvement and serositis manifesting as pericarditis. Similarly, nivolumab and ipilimumab lead to cardiac toxicity, including pericarditis and myocarditis [42, 43].

In the presence of systemic findings, sarcoidosis and amyloidosis should be kept on mind as the causes of pericarditis [44].

Despite explaining multiple reasons about the source of pericarditis, up to 90% of the cases no clear etiology can be established and diagnosis is made as "acute idiopathic pericarditis".

4.2 Epidemiology

The incidence of acute pericarditis is nearly 27.7/100,000 individuals per year. In developed countries, mortality rate of the disease is 1.1%. Acute pericarditis can be developed in all age groups, however, it is common in patients age between 20 and 50 years. Racial predilection is not defined related to disease. Men are more commonly affected than women. Most of the cases with pericarditis is idiopathic. In developed countries the main reasons of the acute pericarditis are viral infections and malignancies. Tuberculosis and HIV infections are the common causes of pericarditis in developing countries [8, 45–48].

4.3 Pathogenesis

Spread of cardiotrophic viruses to the pericardium usually happens via hematogenous way. Thus inflammation and fibrinous changes occur with the infiltration of PMN leukocytes which lead to pericardial effusion. Bacterial pericarditis result from various ways such as contagious spread of infection within the chest via trauma or surgery, spread from infective endocarditis, hematogenous spread of infection or direct inoculation. Spread of tuberculosis pericarditis happens via lymphatic way or contagious spread from a focus of infection in the lung or pleura [6].

4.4 Clinical presentation and diagnosis

Approximately 95% of the cases with acute pericarditis have sharp, retrosternal, and pleuritic pain that radiates into arms, neck, or jaw like acute myocardial infarction (AMI). However, pain in the acute pericarditis has different manifestations from pain due to AMI. It increases in the supine position with inspiration and coughing. It improves by leaning forward and seated position because of reduced pressure on the parietal pericardium. It also respondless to nitrates in opposite to AMI. Chest pain may radiate to shoulders and trapezius ridges which hardens to make differential diagnosis from other causes of life-threatening diseases like aortic dissection or MI [49]. So differential diagnosis should be performed promptly with the diseases angina pectoris, esophagitis, acute gastritis, gastroesophageal reflux disease, AMI, myocardial ischemia, peptic ulcus disease, pleuritis, pneumonia, esophageal spasm, pulmonary embolism, tension pneumothorax, acute aortic dissection, and esophageal rupture [50].

In the literature, predictors of severe illness in patients with acute pericarditis were defined. Major predictors are; fever greater than 38°C, subacute onset, evidence of cardiac tamponade, large pericardial effusion (an echo-free space greater than 20 mm), and ineffective non-steroidal anti-inflammatory drug treatment after 7 days. Minor predictors are immuncompromised state, acute trauma, history of anticoagulant therapy, and elevated cardiac troponin levels [51].

If the etiologic factor is bacterial originated patients may present fever, chills, and leukocytosis whereas gastrointestinal or influenza-like symptoms may present in viral etiology [49].

A pericardial friction rub within auscultation is highly pathognomonic and specific for acute pericarditis. It can be detected 35–85% of the cases according to data of different studies. It is characterized by scratchy, rasping triphasic sound related to friction between pericardial layers during atrial and ventricular systole and early ventricular diastole. The intensity of the sound may increase during auscultation in the position of lean forward. Differential diagnosis between pleural and pericardial rub can be performed by asking the patient to hold the breath while auscultation. According to this physical examination if rub is still present it represents the pericardial rub. Because respiration does not affect pericardial friction rub. It should be kept on mind that despite the sensitivity and diagnostic value of frictional rub, its absence does not rule out the diagnosis [52, 53].

Electrocardiographic findings due to pericardial inflammation can be observed nearly 90% of the individuals with acute pericarditis. Four stages of echocardiographic changes were defined: stage 1: diffuse, concave ST segment elevation, stage 2: ST segment normalize, J point returns to baseline, T wave amplitude begins to decrease, PR segment depression begins to appear, stage 3: symmetric, diffuse T wave invertions, stage 4: changes normalize or T wave inversions may become permanent (**Figure 1**). Beside, Q waves and reciprocal ST segment changes are absent in opposite to AMI [54].

According to European Society of Cardiology 2015 Guidelines, two of four criteria are required to diagnose acute pericarditis [37]. These criteria are;

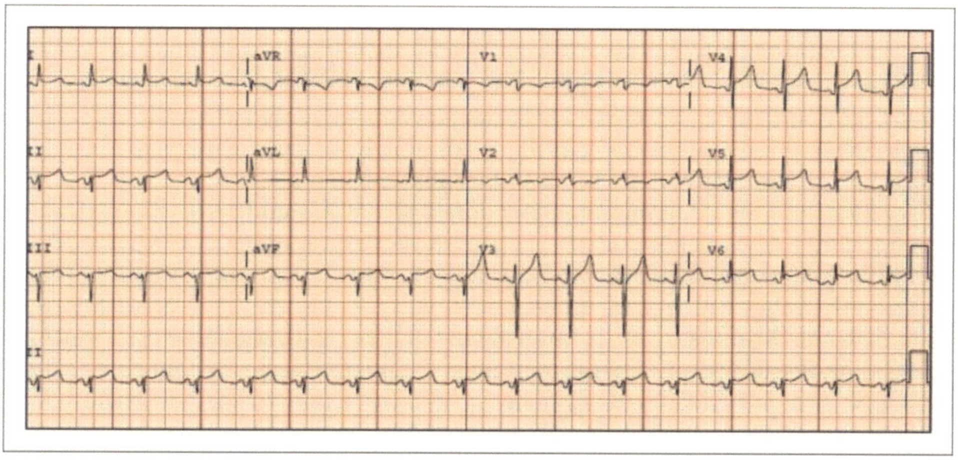

Figure 1.
ECG changes including nearly diffuse, concave-upwards ST-segment elevation, and PR-segment depressions in acute pericarditis.

1. Pericardial chest pain

2. Pericardial frictional rubs

3. New widespread ST segment elevation or PR segment depression on ECG

4. New or worsening pericardial effusion

In addition to anamnesis, physical examination and electrocardiographic findings supportive findings like chest X-ray, cardiac computed tomography, magnetic resonance imaging, basic metabolic panel, complete blood count, erythrocyte sedimentation rate (ESR), C reactive protein (CRP), troponin I and creatine kinase levels can be used in the evaluation of the disease [55]. Chest radiography is useful to detect the abnormalities related to lungs and mediastinum, especially for pericardial effusion. WBC count, CRP levels, and ESR are usually elevated. Long duration of elevated CRP levels (usually normalizes in 85% of the patients within 2 weeks after treatment) suggests continued inflammation and requires prolonged therapy. Troponin I levels can be elevated up to 50% of patients in association with epicardial inflammation in oppose to myocyte necrosis seen in AMI. This elevation is transient and resolves within 1–2 weeks without adverse prognosis. Elevation of CK-MB can accompany or not [49].

In selected patients viral seromarkers, blood culture and tests for tuberculosis like PPD or quentiferon tuberculosis assay can be performed. If there is a suspicion of opportunistic infection, HIV testing should be obtained because of strong correlation between tuberculosis and fungal infections and immune-suppressed state. Further studies such as anti nuclear antibody or tests toward a systemic disease (systemic lupus erythamosus, sarcoidosis ...) may be done [56].

Despite disadvantages like ionizing radiation and frequent requirement of intravenous contrast material, CT is very useful for evaluating pericardial anatomy, anatomic variants and pericardial abnormalities. On CT scan of patients with acute pericarditis thickening of the pericardium with smooth margins and intense early contrast enhancement with various amounts of effusion can be detected [57].

Cardiac MRI is another method for the evaluation of the pericardium. It has good spatial and temporal resolution with highly reproducible measurement and does not expose radiation to the patients. Smooth and thickened pericardial images suggest acute or subacute pericarditis whereas irregular and thickened pericardium indicates chronic pericarditis, tumors, metastasis, or fibrosis. It also identifies loculated or localized pericardial effusions with its nature [58].

Two diagnostic imaging methods mentioned above (CT and MRI) should be considered as further imaging modalities in patients with underlying etiologies such as systemic inflammatory diseases, neoplasms, renal diseases, and tuberculosis. Routine trans-thoracic echocardiography is recommended in all patients with acute pericarditis as a first-line diagnostic tool. It can be used to detect the pericardial effusion and its hemodynamic effects on cardiac structures if constrictive pericarditis or cardiac tamponade is suspected (**Figure 2**). It also gives opportunity to exclude AMI by the evaluation of the abnormalities in wall motion [59].

If there is a suspicion of tuberculosis, neoplastic or purulent pericarditis, or an effusion refractory to treatment leads to cardiac tamponade or hemodynamic compromise, then pericardiocentesis and if possible biopsy of the pericardium are indicated. Symptomatic or large pericardial effusion refractory to treatment also requires pericardiocentesis [50]. In a study designed by Permanyer it is emphasized that rate of pericardial tamponade differs 5–15% of patients with acute idiopathic pericarditis and up to 60% of those with purulent, neoplasm or tuberculosis pericarditis [60].

Two dimensional and M-mode Doppler echocardiography is specific, non-invasive, sensitive, and easily available technique and the gold standard for the diagnosis of pericardial effusion. Small amounts of pericardial fluid may be physiologic and detected during ventricular systole. If it is over 50 mL en echo-free space persists throughout the cardiac cycle. Small effusion was initially detected over the posterobasal left ventricle, as the volume increases it spreads anterior, lateral, and behind parts of the left atrium. "Swinging heart" is a possible sign of pericardial tamponade due to large pericardial effusion [61].

Pericardial effusion analysis can help for the diagnosis of neoplastic and infectious effusions. Tumor markers and cytology should be performed in suspicion of

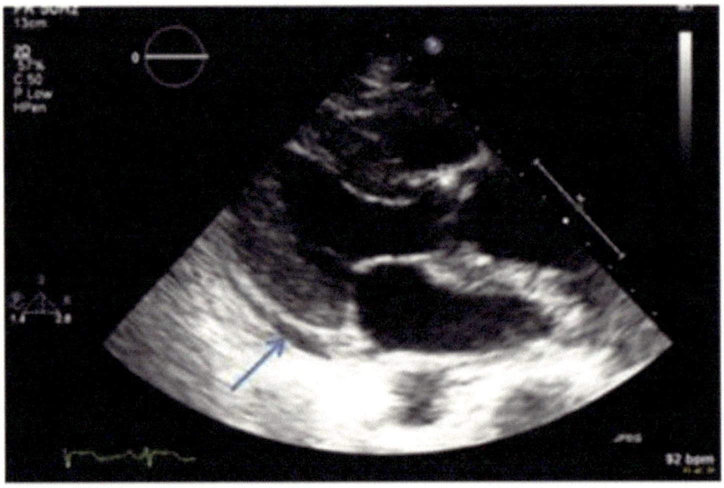

Figure 2.
Echocardiogram showing acute pericarditis with small pericardial effusion.

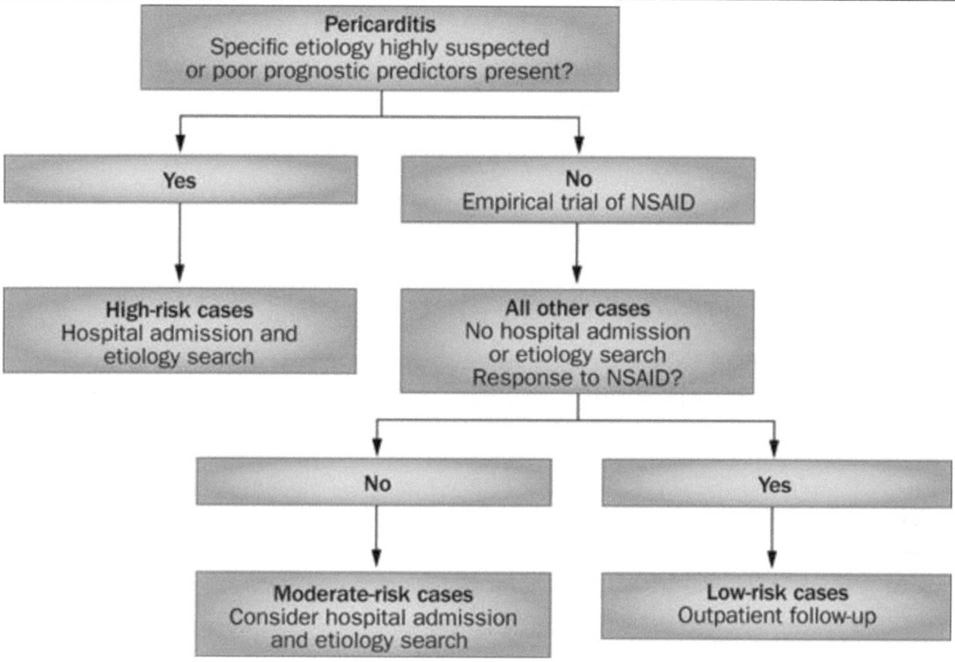

Table 1.
A summarized perspective for the diagnosis and management of pericarditis [63].

malignancy. Pericardial fluid culture should performed at least three times with the blood culture in suspected bacterial infections [62].

Diagnosis and management of pericarditis was summarized in **Table 1**.

4.5 Treatment

Exercise restriction is recommended therapy for all patients during the symptoms and at least 3 months for athletes. Ibuprofen can be started at 3 × 600 mg/day for 1 or 2 weeks with proton pump inhibitor and dose can be decreased to 400 mg/week when the inflammatory markers become normalized in acute pericarditis [37]. In patients with a history or significant risk factors for coronary artery disease (CAD), aspirin may be used instead of ibuprofen at a dose of 900 mg/day for 1–2 weeks and dose can be decreased to 600 mg/week when the symptoms resolve and inflammation markers normalize. Colchicine treatment requires a careful follow up the patients because of increased risk of incessant or recurrent pericarditis. If appropriately used with pay attention to narrow therapeutic index of the drug, it can be safe. Potential drug interactions and comorbidities of the patients also be kept on mind while prescribing the drug [64]. If underlying autoimmune rheumatic diseases lead to acute pericarditis or there is a contraindication to NSAIDs or colchicines, corticosteroids can be used. Although they are initially effective, they may promote recurrence and attenuate the efficiency of colchicines if used first-line. In the state of idiopathic pericarditis steroids should only be used as adjuvant therapy if there is a recurrence after a trial of NSAIDs and colchicine. Duration of the steroid treatment is 4 weeks if the inflammation markers normalize and symptoms resolve, and doses must be tapered slowly to avoid adrenal insufficiency [31, 65].

For the patients failing first-line therapy with NSAIDs and colchicine or second-line therapy with NSAIDs, steroids, and colchicines, third-line therapeutic approach is possible. This modality includes azathiprine, intravenous immunoglobulin, and an interleukin 1 beta antagonist called anakinra. Surgical pericardiectomy is the last option and rarely required in clinical practice especially to whom has previous cardiac surgery and/or features of constrictive pericarditis [64].

4.6 Miscellaneous facts about acute pericarditis

4.6.1 COVID-19 and acute pericarditis

COVID-19 disease primarily affects respiratory system however, cardiac involvement such as heart failure, myocardial infarction, arrhythmias, endocarditis, myocarditis, and pericarditis were reported nearly 10% of the patients with COVID-19. Although pericarditis was diagnosed in the minority of the cases with COVID-19, accompanied pericardial effusion and cardiac tamponade were observed in some of those patients [66]. Various hypothesis about cardiac involvement due to COVID-19 are mentioned in the literature. One of them emphasized that direct SARS-CoV-2 effects could be the result of cardiac injuries. ACE 2 receptors highly expressed in lung and heart plays a main role in the mechanism of the inflammation [67]. Macrophage-induced inflammation is the other hypothesis for cardiac complication in patients with COVID-19. Activation of macrophages results in release of massive amounts of cytokine which leads to endothelial activation, expression of adhesion molecules for inflammatory cell infiltration and vascular inflammation [68].

Patients with COVID-19 had pericardial effusion up to 27%, although, severity of effusion was mild in the majority of the cases. In addition, pericarditis is associated with high mortality rates and onset of new cardiac complications such as atrial fibrillation and heart failure [69].

4.6.2 Acute pericarditis after chemotherapy

Relationship between high-dose chemotherapy and acute pericarditis was suggested in the literature. Despite unknown mechanism, opportunistic infections, direct toxic or immunological drug-related mechanisms may play a role in this clinical situation [70].

Conflict of interest

The authors declare no conflict of interest.

DOI: http://dx.doi.org/10.5772/intechopen.109354

Author details

Erhan Hafiz[1] and Ozgur Altinbas[2*]

1 Department of Cardiovascular Surgery, Gaziantep University, Gaziantep, Turkey

2 Vocational School of Health Services, Gaziantep University, Gaziantep, Turkey

*Address all correspondence to: ozgur_altinbas@yahoo.com

IntechOpen

© 2023 The Author(s). Licensee IntechOpen. This chapter is distributed under the terms of the Creative Commons Attribution License (http://creativecommons.org/licenses/by/3.0), which permits unrestricted use, distribution, and reproduction in any medium, provided the original work is properly cited.

References

[1] Rodriguez ER, Tan CD. Structure and anatomy of the human pericardium. Progress in Cardiovascular Diseases. 2017;**59**(4):327-340

[2] Dusting GJ, Nolan RD, Woodman OL, Martin TJ. Prostacyclin produced by the pericardium and its influence on coronary vascular tone. The American Journal of Cardiology. 1983;**52**(2):28-35

[3] Mebazaa A, Wetzel RC, Dodd JM, Redmond EM, Maeda SK, Maistre G, et al. Potential paracrine role of the pericardium in the regulation of cardiac function. Cardiovascular Research. 1998;**40**(2):332-342

[4] Dudzinski DM, Mak GS, Hung JW. Pericardial diseases. Current Problems in Cardiology. 2012;**37**(3):75-118

[5] Little WC, Freeman GL. Pericardial disease. Circulation. 2006;**113**(12):1622-1632

[6] Khandaker MH, Espinosa RE, Nishimura RA, Sinak LJ, Hayes SN, Meldeni RM, et al. Pericardial disease: Diagnosis and management. Mayo Clinic Proceedings. 2010;**85**(6):572-593

[7] Mayosi BM, Burgess LJ, Doubell AF. Tuberculous pericarditis. Circulation. 2005;**112**(23):3608-3616

[8] Kytö V, Sipila J, Rautava P. Clinical profile and influences on outcomes in patients hospitalized for acute pericarditis. Circulation. 2014;**130**(18):1601-1606

[9] Poorsattar SP, Maus TM. Pericardium. In: Maus TM, Tainter CR, editors. Essential Echocardiography. Cham: Springer; 2022

[10] Volpe JK, Makaryus AN. Anatomy, Thorax, Heart and Pericardial Cavity. [Updated Jul 31, 2021]. In: StatPearls [Internet]. Treasure Island (FL): StatPearls Publishing; 2022

[11] Rehman I, Nassereddin A, Rehman A. Anatomy, Thorax, Pericardium. [Updated Jul 27, 2021]. In: StatPearls [Internet]. Treasure Island (FL): StatPearls Publishing; 2022

[12] Ozan H. Anatomy of the pericardium. Turkiye Klinikleri Cardiology - Special Topics. 2009;**2**(6):1-5

[13] Vogiatzidis K, Zarogiannis SG, Aidonidis I, Solenov EI, Molydas PA, Gourgoulianis KI, et al. Physiology of pericardial fluid production and drainage. Frontiers in Physiology. 2015;**6**:1-6

[14] Ishihara T, Ferrans VJ, Jones M, Boyce SW, Kawanami O, Roberts WC. Histologic and ultrastructural features of normal human parietal pericardium. The American Journal of Cardiology. 1980;**46**(5):744-753

[15] Hoit BD. Pathophysiology of the pericardium. Progress in Cardiovascular Diseases. 2017;**59**(5):341-348

[16] Khandaker MH, Espinosa RE, Nishimura RA, Sinak LJ, Hayes SN, Melduni RM, et al. Pericardial disease: Diagnose and management. Mayo Clinic Proceedings. 2010;**85**(6):572-593

[17] JLAd S, Greguolo C, JFF J, Paiva AN, Trad HS, TTd A. Partial congenital absence of pericardium. Revista Brasileira de Cardiologia Invasiva. 2012;**20**:435-437

[18] Shah AB, Krozon I. Congenital defects of the pericardium. European Heart Journal. 2015;**16**(8):821-827

[19] Nayak K, Shetty RK, Vivek G, Pai UM. Pericardial cyst: A benign anomaly. Case Reports. 2012;**2012**:1-2

[20] Barcin C, Kabul HK. Pericardial tamponade. Turkiye Klinikleri Cardiology - Special Topics. 2009;**2**(6):32-39

[21] Duran A, Ocak T, Uyeturk U, Erdem A, Onder H, Maltas MS. Cardiac tamponade with primary certain non-malignancy in clinic. Konuralp Medical Journal. 2014;**6**(2):58-60

[22] Pacha HM, Soud M, Alraies MC. Beyond Beck's triad: A rare cause of cardiac tamponade and hemoptysis. The Ochsner Journal. 2018;**18**(3):271-273

[23] Turhan S, Tutar E. Acute Cardiac Tamponade. Türk Yoğun Bakım Dergisi. 2004;**4**(2):105-112

[24] Adegbala O, Olagoke O, Adejumo A, Akintoye E, Oluwole A, Alebna P, et al. Incidence and outcomes of cardiac tamponade in patients undergoing cardiac resynchronization therapy. International Journal of Cardiology. 2018;**272**:137-141

[25] Imazio M, Mayosi BM, Brucato A, Markel G, Trinchero R, Spodick DH, et al. Triage and management of pericardial effusion. Journal of Cardiovascular Medicine. 2010;**11**(12):928-935

[26] Sagrista SJ, Merce J, Permanyer MG, Soler J. Clinical clues to the causes of large pericardial effusions. The American Journal of Medicine. 2000;**109**:95-101

[27] Alerhand S, Carter JM. What echocardiographic findings suggest a pericardial effusion is causing tamponade? The American Journal of Emergency Medicine. 2019;**37**(2):321-326

[28] Casares AP, Cesar S, Garcia LB, Toledo JS. Echocardiographic evaluation of pericardial effusion and cardiac tamponade. Frontiers in Pediatrics. 2017;**5**:79-88

[29] Imazio M. Pericardial involvement in systemic inflammatory diseases. Heart. 2011;**97**:1882-1892

[30] Imazio M, Brucato A, Trinchero R, Spodick DH, Adler Y. Colchicine for pericarditis: Hype or hope? European Heart Journal. 2009;**30**:532-539

[31] Imazio M, Brucato A, Cumetti D, Trinchero R. Corticosteroids for recurrent pericarditis: High versus low doses: A nonrandomized observation. Circulation. 2008;**118**:667-671

[32] Vianello F, Cinetto F, Cavraro M, Battsiti A, Castelli M, Imbergamo S, et al. Azathioprine in isolated recurrent pericarditis: A single center experience. International Journal of Cardiology. 2011;**47**:477-478

[33] Nishimura RA. Constrictive pericarditis in the modern era: A diagnostic dilemma. Heart. 2010;**86**:619-623

[34] Ling LH, Oh JK, Schaff HV, Danielson GK, Mahoney DW, Seward JB, et al. Constrictive pericarditis in the modern era: Evolving clinical spectrum and impact outcome after pericardiectomy. Circulation. 1999;**100**:1380-1386

[35] Maisch B. Management of pericarditis and pericardial effusion, constrictive pericarditis and effusive-constrictive pericarditis. Herz. 2018;**43**(7):663-678

[36] Fardman A, Charron P, Imazio M, Adler Y. European guidelines on pericardial diseases: A focused review of novel aspects. Current Cardiology Reports. 2016;**18**(5):46-55

[37] Adler Y, Charron P. The ESC guidelines on the diagnosis and management of pericardial diseases. European Heart Journal. 2015;**36**(42):2873-2874

[38] Petcu CP, Dilof R, Bataiosu C, Petca D. Purulent pericardial effusions with pericardial tamponade – diagnosis and treatment issues. Current Health Sciences. 2013;**39**(1):53-56

[39] Oladele RO, Ayanlowo OO, Richardson MD, Denning DW. Histoplasmosis in Africa: An emerging or a neglected disease? PLoS Neglected Tropical Diseases. 2018;**12**(1):e0006046

[40] McCague A, Serio K, Leibe J. Delayed-onset pericarditis in non penetrating blunt force trauma: A case report. Trauma Cases and Reviews. 2016;**2**(3):1-3

[41] Jaworska WM, Abramczuk E, Hryniewiecki T. Postcardiac injury syndrome. Medical Science Monitor. 2011;**17**(11):13-14

[42] Katz U, Zandman-Goddard G. Drug-induced lupus: An update. Autoimmunity Reviews. 2010;**10**(1):46-50

[43] Altan M, Toki MI, Gettinger SN, Carvajal-Hausdorf DE, Zugazagoitia J, Sinard JH, et al. Immune checkpoint inhibitor-associated pericarditis. Journal of Thoracic Oncology. 2019;**14**(6):1102-1108

[44] Wyplosz B, Marijon E, Dougados J, Pouchot J. Sarcoidosis: An unusual cause of acute pericarditis. Acta Cardiologica. 2010;**65**(1):83-84

[45] Ariyarajah V, Spodick DH. Acute pericarditis. Cardiology in Review. 2007;**15**(1):24-30

[46] Troughton RW, Asher CR, Klein AL. Pericarditis. Lancet. 2004;**363**(9410):717-727

[47] Sagristà-Sauleda J, Permanyer-Miralda G, Soler-Soler J. Tuberculosis pericarditis: Ten year experience with a prospective protocol for diagnosis and treatment. Journal of the American College of Cardiology. 1988;**11**(4):724-728

[48] Chen Y, Brennessel D, Walters J, Johnson M, Rosner F, Raza M. Human immunodeficiency virus-associated pericardial effusion: Report of 40 cases and review of literature. American Heart Journal. 1999;**137**(3):516-521

[49] Matthew JS, Bepko J, White M. Acute pericarditis: Diagnosis and management. American Family Physician. 2014;**89**(7):553-560

[50] Gibbons RJ, Chatterjee K, Daley J. ACC/AHA/ACP-ASIM guidelines for the management of patients with chronic stable angina: A report of the American College of Cardiology/American Heart Association Task Force on Practice Guidelines (Committee on Management of Patients with Chronic Stable Angina) [published corrections appear in J Am Coll Cardiol. 1999;34(1):314, and J Am Coll Cardiol. 2001;38(1):296]. Journal of the American College of Cardiology. 1999;**33**(7):2092-2197

[51] Imazio M, Cecchi E, Demichelis B, Ierna S, Demarie D, Ghisio A, et al. Indicators of poor prognosis of acute pericarditis. Circulation. 2007;**115**(21):2739-2744

[52] Lange RA, Hillis LD. Clinical practice: Acute pericarditis. The New England Journal of Medicine. 2004;**351**(21):2195-2202

[53] Zayas R, Angurita M, Torres F, Gimenez D, Bergillos F, Ruiz M, et al. Incidence of specific etiology and role of methods for spesific etiologic diagnosis of primary acute pericarditis.

The American Journal of Cardiology. 1995;**75**(5):378-382

[54] Ginzton LE, Laks MM. The differential diagnosis of acute pericarditis from the normal variant: New electrocardiographic criteria. Circulation. 1982;**65**(5):1004-1009

[55] Imazio M, Spodick DH, Brucato A, Trinchero R, Markel G, Adler Y. Diagnostic issues in the clinical management of pericarditis. International Journal of Clinical Practice. 2010;**64**(10):1384-1392

[56] Imazio M, Spodick DH, Brucato A, Trinchero R, Adler Y. Controversial issues in the management of pericardial diseases. Circulation. 2010;**121**(7):916-928

[57] Rajiah P, Kanne JP. Computed tomography of the pericardium and pericardial disease. Journal of Cardiovascular Computed Tomography. 2010;**4**(1):3-18

[58] Maksimovic R, Dill T, Seferovic PM, Ristic AD, Alter P, Simeunovic DS, et al. Magnetic resonance imaging in pericardial diseases. Herz. 2006;7:708-711

[59] Niraj S, Shah AB, Coplan N, Kronzon I. Acute pericarditis. Progress in Cardiovascular Diseases. 2017;**59**(4):349-359

[60] Permanyer-Miralda G. Acute pericardial disease: Approach to the aetiologic diagnosis. Heart. 2004;**90**(3):252-254

[61] Jung HO. Pericardial effusion and pericardiocentesis: Role of echocardiography. Korean Circulation Journal. 2012;**42**(11):725-734

[62] Imazio M, Adler Y. Management of pericardial effusion. European Heart Journal. 2013;**34**(16):1186-1197

[63] Imazio M, Brucato A, Trinchero R, et al. Diagnosis and management of pericardial diseases. Nature Reviews. Cardiology. 2009;**6**:743-751

[64] Ismail TF. Acute pericarditis: Update on diagnosis and management. Clinical Medicine. 2020;**20**(1):48-51

[65] Artom G, Koren-Morag N, Spodick DH, et al. Pretreatment with corticosteroids attenuates the efficacy of colchicine in preventing recurrent pericarditis: A multi-centre all-case analysis. European Heart Journal. 2005;**26**:723-727

[66] Singh A, Nguyen L, Everest S, Shastri P, Alemu RH. Acute pericarditis secondary to COVID-19 infection. Cureus. 2021;**13**(12):e20709

[67] Aghagoli G, Gallo MB, Soliman LB, Sellke PW. Cardiac involvement in COVID-19 patients: Risk factors, predictors, and complications: A review. Journal of Cardiac Surgery. 2020;**35**:1302-1305

[68] Su YB, Kuo MJ, Lin TY, Chien CS, Yang YP, Chou SJ, et al. Cardiovascular manifestation and treatment in COVID-19. Journal of the Chinese Medical Association : JCMA. 2020;**83**:704-709

[69] Lazar M, Barbu EC, Chitu CE, Anghel AM, Niculae CM, Manea ED, et al. Pericardial involvement in severe COVID-19 patients. Medicina. 2022;**58**:1093-1101

[70] Bock J, Doenitz A, Andreesen R, Reichle A, Hennemann B. Pericarditis after high-dose chemotherapy: More frequent than expected? Onkologie. 2006;**29**(7):321-325

Chapter 2

PET Imaging of Infection

Christopher J. Palestro

Abstract

Nuclear medicine has played an important part in the diagnosis of infection for 50 years. Gallium-67 citrate was one of the first radionuclides used for diagnosing and localizing infection. The development of techniques for radiolabeling leukocytes and monitoring their migration to foci of infection was a significant advance. More recently, investigators have worked on developing positron-emitting radiopharmaceuticals for diagnosing infection. Positron emission tomography (PET) provides high-resolution three-dimensional images, facilitating precise localization of radiopharmaceutical uptake. Semiquantitative analysis could facilitate the differentiation of infectious from noninfectious conditions and could be used to monitor treatment response. Not surprisingly, the first PET agent investigated was fluorine 18-fluorodeoxyglucose (^{18}F-FDG). Although ^{18}F-FDG has proved to be invaluable for diagnosing infection, it is not specific, and also accumulates in neoplasms, and noninfectious inflammatory conditions. Considerable effort has been devoted to developing PET radiopharmaceuticals that are specific, or at least more specific than ^{18}F-FDG, for infection. Investigators have explored the potential of leukocytes labeled in vitro with various PET radiopharmaceuticals, gallium-68 citrate, gallium-68 labeled peptides, iodine-124 fialuridine, and ^{18}F-fluorodeoxysorbitol. This chapter reviews the role of ^{18}F-FDG for diagnosing infection and monitoring treatment response and other PET agents whose potential for diagnosing infection has been studied.

Keywords: cardiovascular infections, ^{18}F-FDG, ^{18}F-FDS, ^{124}FIAU, FUO, gallium, osteomyelitis, sarcoid, spondylodiscitis, tuberculosis, zirconium

1. Introduction

Infection is a major cause of patient morbidity and mortality throughout the world. The diagnosis of infection can be challenging and imaging studies are often used for confirmation and localization. Radiological tests, such as x-rays, ultrasonography, computed tomography, and magnetic resonance imaging, reflect structural alterations in tissues and organs produced by a combination of the infection and the host's response to the infection. Structural changes take time to evolve and there is a delay between the molecular events of the disease process itself and the appearance of structural changes on radiologic imaging. Nuclear medicine imaging agents can be taken up directly by cells, tissues, and organs, or can be attached to native substances that then migrate to an inflammatory focus. These agents reflect physiological changes in the inflammatory process and can identify abnormalities before the development of structural changes [1]. For many years, the single photon emitting radiopharmaceuticals, gallium-67 citrate, and *in vitro* labeled leukocytes were the mainstay of nuclear medicine imaging of infection. Positron emission tomography (PET) has several advantages over single photon imaging. PET provides high-resolution three-dimensional images of the whole body facilitating precise localization of radiopharmaceutical uptake. Semiquantitative analysis could facilitate the differentiation of infectious from noninfectious conditions and could be useful for monitoring response to treatment. In view of the advantages of PET over single photon imaging as well as the proliferation of clinical PET over the past 25 years, it is not surprising that investigators have turned their attention to developing PET radiopharmaceuticals for diagnosing infection. The first and most extensively studied of these agents is fluorine-18 fluorodeoxyglucose (^{18}F-FDG). Developed primarily for oncology, ^{18}F-FDG uptake in inflammation was soon recognized. While such uptake could confound study interpretation in patients with tumors, the possibility of ^{18}F-FDG for imaging infection was exploited [2]. The potential of human leukocytes labeled *in vitro* with ^{18}F-FDG, copper-64 (^{64}Cu), and zirconium-89 (^{89}Zr) for imaging infection has also been investigated. Other PET agents that have been studied include gallium-68 (^{68}Ga) citrate, iodine-124 (^{124}I)-filauridine, fluorine-18 fluorodeoxysorbitol (^{18}F-FDS), and ^{68}Ga labeled peptides.

2. ^{18}F-FDG

Cellular uptake of fluorodeoxyglucose, which is a structural analog of 2-deoxyglucose, is governed by three mechanisms: passive diffusion, active transport by a Na1-dependent glucose transporter (GLUT), and *via* GLUT-1 through GLUT-13 transporters. Once inside the cell, it is phosphorylated to 2'-FDG-6 phosphate by the hexokinase enzyme. Unlike glucose-6-phosphate, 2'-FDG-6 phosphate is not a substrate for the enzymes of the glycolytic pathway or the pentose–phosphate shunt. It is trapped intracellularly but is not metabolized, and does not diffuse back into the extracellular space [3].

The normal distribution of ^{18}F-FDG includes the brain, myocardium, and urinary tract. Thymic uptake, particularly in children, has been observed. Gastric and bowel activity are variable. Liver, spleen, and bone marrow uptake generally are low-grade (**Figure 1**) [4]. The small ^{18}F-FDG molecule enters poorly perfused areas rapidly, so imaging can be performed within 1–2 hours after administration. Skeletal uptake usually normalizes within 3–4 months after trauma or surgery, and degenerative bone

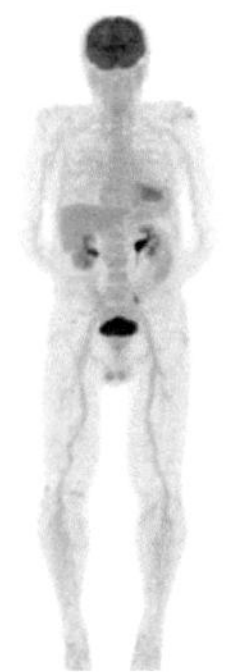

Figure 1.
Normal ^{18}F-FDG maximum intensity projection image. There is brain, myocardial, liver, spleen, and urinary tract activity. Faint bone marrow uptake is present.

changes ordinarily show only mildly increased uptake, which are advantageous when musculoskeletal infection is a concern [5]. Over the past two decades, ^{18}F-FDG has assumed an increasingly important role in molecular imaging of infection.

2.1 Musculoskeletal infection

^{18}F-FDG has proved to be very useful for diagnosing osteomyelitis (**Figure 2**). In one systematic review, ^{18}F-FDG PET had a pooled sensitivity of 0.92 (95% CI: 0.87–0.96) and a pooled specificity of 0.92 (95% CI: 0.87–0.96) for the diagnosis of osteomyelitis, for a positive likelihood ratio of 9.77 (95% CI: 5.99–15.95) and a negative likelihood ratio of 0.12 (95% CI: 0.07–0.20). The area under the summary receiver operating characteristics curve was 0.97 [6]. In another systematic review, ^{18}F-FDG PET had a pooled sensitivity of 0.96 (95% CI: 0.88–0.99) and a pooled specificity of 0.91 (95% CI: 0.81–0.95) for diagnosing chronic osteomyelitis [7].

2.1.1 Spondylodiscitis

The role of ^{18}F-FDG in the diagnosis of spondylodiscitis has been extensively studied. The pooled sensitivity and specificity of ^{18}F-FDG PET/PET-CT were 97% and 88% in one meta-analysis [8]. In another meta-analysis, the pooled sensitivity was 94.8% and the pooled specificity was 91.4% (**Figure 3**) [9] . In intraindividual comparisons, ^{18}F-FDG has outperformed bone and gallium-67 scintigraphy both alone and in combination [10, 11].

Postoperative spondylodiscitis often has an indolent, nonspecific presentation. Prompt diagnosis is imperative because a delay may lead to involvement of the bone, epidural space, and paravertebral soft tissues, and may necessitate hardware removal, which can lead to instability and pseudoarthrosis [12]. In a meta-analysis of ^{18}F-FDG for diagnosing postoperative spondylodiscitis, the summary AUC for spondylodiscitis was 0.92 in patients with versus 0.98 in patients without spinal hardware. False-positive results were more common in patients with than in patients without hardware (12.8% vs. 7%), presumably due to hardware-induced aseptic inflammation. Performing PET/CT rather than PET alone reduces hardware-associated false-positive results [8]. Analyzing uptake patterns may facilitate the differentiation between aseptic inflammation and infection. Confluent increased ^{18}F-FDG uptake in soft tissue and bone immediately adjacent to the hardware at multiple contiguous levels

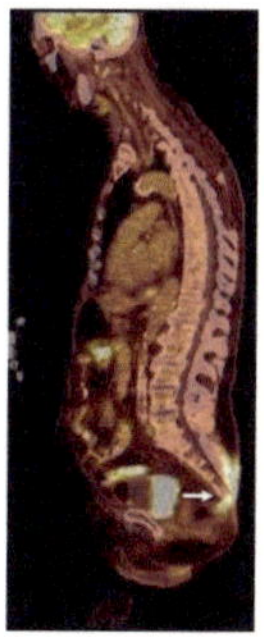

Figure 2.
Sacral osteomyelitis. There is ^{18}F-FDG uptake in a sacral decubitus ulcer extending into the distal sacrum (arrow).

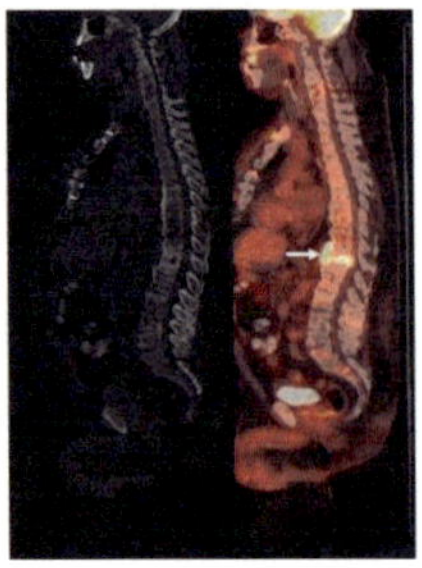

Figure 3.
Spondylodiscitis. There is abnormal ^{18}F-FDG activity in the T12-L1 vertebrae corresponding to erosive changes on the CT component, with extension into the prevertebral space (arrow).

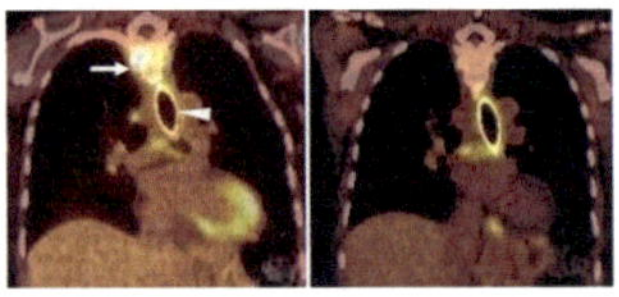

Figure 4.
Spondylodiscitis thoracic spine. On the pretreatment ^{18}F-FDG PET/CT (left) there is intense uptake in the T2-T3 vertebrae (arrow). On the posttreatment study, performed about 3 months later, the abnormal uptake had resolved. Persistent esophageal activity (arrowhead) was thought to be secondary to a foreign body reaction or metastatic disease in this patient with esophageal carcinoma (reproduced with permission from Seminars in Nuclear Medicine: Raghavan M, Palestro CJ: Imaging spondylodiscitis: an update. 53:152-166. DOI: 10.1053/j.semnuclmed.2022.11.005).

is suggestive of infection, while focal uptake adjacent to one or two hooks, screws, or anchors, usually at the upper or lower aspects of the spinal hardware is more suggestive of noninfectious complications [13].

^{18}F-FDG may be useful for monitoring treatment response in spondylodiscitis (**Figure 4**). Some investigators have reported that changes in standardized uptake value (SUV) reliably differentiate responders from nonresponders, while other investigators have observed that changes in uptake patterns are useful for monitoring treatment response [14–19].

2.1.2 Diabetic pedal osteomyelitis

Because diabetics can have a significant foot infection with few signs or symptoms and without mounting a systemic inflammatory response, the diagnosis of osteomyelitis can easily be overlooked [20]. Molecular imaging has always had an important role in the workup of these patients and data indicate that ^{18}F-FDG is useful in this population. In one meta-analysis, the pooled sensitivity and specificity of ^{18}F-FDG were 74% and 91%, respectively [21].

In another meta-analysis, the pooled sensitivity and specificity of ^{18}F-FDG were 89% and 92%, respectively, which was similar to the pooled sensitivity and specificity of ^{99m}Tc-labeled leukocyte scintigraphy: 91% and 92%, respectively [22].

2.1.3 Periprosthetic joint infection

In a systematic review the pooled sensitivity and specificity of ^{18}F-FDG-PET for diagnosing lower extremity periprosthetic joint infection (PJI) were 86% (95%

CI: 82–90%) and 86% (95% CI: 83–89%), respectively [23]. In another systematic review, the pooled sensitivity and specificity of ^{18}F-FDG-PET for lower extremity PJI were 82.1% (95% CI: 68.0–90.8%) and 86.6% (95% CI: 79.7–91.4%), respectively [24]. The authors noted that caution is warranted because results of individual studies were heterogeneous and could not be fully explored. These limitations are borne out by the inconsistent results reported in individual investigations over the years [25]. Different test probabilities, the inability to discriminate between infection and aseptic inflammation, and a lack of standardized interpretative criteria are obstacles to incorporating ^{18}F-FDG-PET into the routine diagnostic imaging workup for PJI (**Figure 5**) [26].

Data on ^{18}F-FDG for diagnosing PJI of shoulder arthroplasties are scant. In an investigation of 86 patients with suspected chronic PJI of the shoulder, the sensitivity and specificity of ^{18}F-FDG PET/CT were 14% (3/22) and 91% (58/64), respectively [27].

2.2 Cardiovascular infections

The term cardiovascular infection encompasses a wide range of infections, including endocarditis, cardiac implantable electronic device (CIED), and prosthetic vascular graft infections. Diagnosis of these often life-threatening conditions can be challenging and ^{18}F-FDG can play an important role in their diagnosis.

2.2.1 Infective endocarditis

Infective endocarditis (IE) is a life-threatening infection. In spite of advances in diagnosis and treatment, patients with IE still have high rates of morbidity and mortality. The diagnosis is based on modified Duke's criteria that classify patients into three categories: definite, possible, and rejected IE. The overall sensitivity of modified Duke's criteria is approximately 80% [28, 29].

^{18}F-FDG is a useful adjunct for diagnosing IE with a pooled sensitivity and specificity of 61% and 88%, respectively (**Figure 6**). It is especially useful in the setting of prosthetic heart valves. False-negative results are associated with lesions below the limits of res olution of current systems and antibiotic treatment for more than 1 week prior to imaging. False positive results can occur with postoperative inflammation during the first 2 months after implantation and in the presence of severe prosthetic valve thrombosis [30, 31].

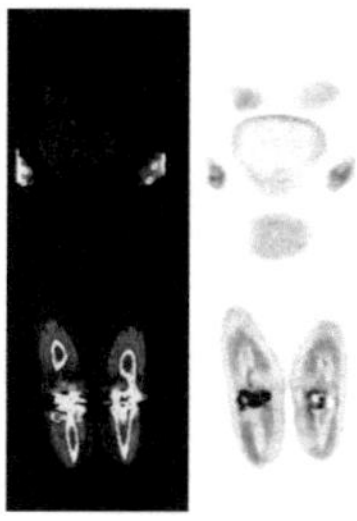

Figure 5.
Asymptomatic knee arthroplasties. There is intense periprosthetic ^{18}F-FDG around the right knee arthroplasty and to lesser extent around the left knee arthroplasty. The inability to be able to consistently discriminate between periprosthetic infection and aseptic inflammation, is a significant disadvantage of ^{18}F-FDG.

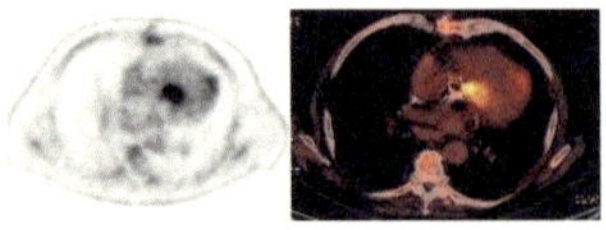

Figure 6.
Infective endocarditis prosthetic aortic valve. ^{18}F-FDG is especially useful for diagnosing infective endocarditis in patients with prosthetic heart valves.

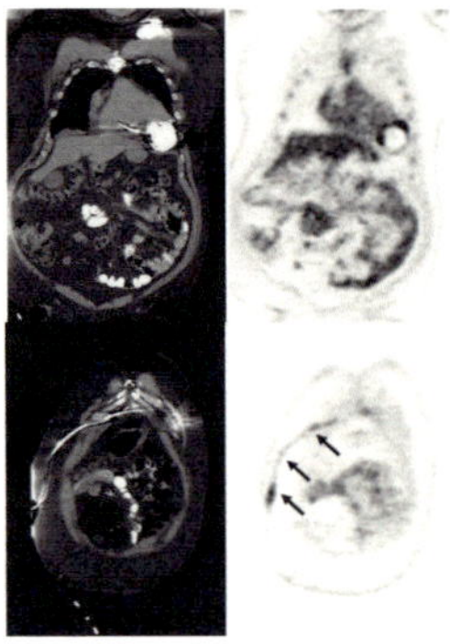

Figure 7.
Infected left ventricular assist device and driveline. There is abnormal ^{18}F-FDG accumulation around the device (top) and driveline (bottom, arrows).

2.2.2 Cardiac implantable electronic device infections

CIEDs, such as permanent pacemakers, cardioverter-defibrillators, and cardiac resynchronization systems, have become increasingly important in the management of cardiac disease. The number of devices implanted has increased over time, especially in older patients with more comorbidities, leading to higher infection rates [32].

^{18}F-FDG is useful for diagnosing CIED infections (**Figure 7**). Besides diagnosing pacemaker pocket infection, ^{18}F-FDG delineates the extent of infection and improves the diagnostic accuracy of the modified Duke's criteria for CIED infection. It is useful for diagnosing left ventricular assist device infection, determining extent of infection, and monitoring treatment response [33–36]. In a meta-analysis of nearly five hundred patients, the pooled sensitivity of ^{18}F-FDG PET/CT for diagnosing CIED infection was 83% and the pooled specificity was 89%. For diagnosing pocket infection, pooled sensitivity and specificity were 96% and 97%, respectively. The test was less sensitive for lead infection and CIED-IE with pooled sensitivity and specificity of 76% and 83%, respectively [37].

2.2.3 Prosthetic vascular graft infections

Although prosthetic vascular graft infections are infrequent, they are associated with high morbidity and sometimes, mortality. Underlying comorbidities increase risk of infection and infection-related complications, such as sepsis, enteric fistulae, spread of infection to other sites, and death [38].

^{18}F-FDG accurately diagnoses prosthetic vascular graft infection, with sensitivity and specificity ranging from 88% to 100% [39, 40]. It is important to be cognizant of the fact that these grafts can incite a foreign-body inflammatory response that can lead to increased ^{18}F-FDG uptake in the absence of infection. Familiarity with typical ^{18}F-FDG uptake patterns associated with infection and foreign body reaction is important. Vascular graft infection generally presents as focal or heterogeneously increased ^{18}F-FDG uptake that projects over the vessel on the CT component of the examination (**Figure 8**). In contrast, the aseptic foreign body reaction presents as linear, diffuse, and homogeneous uptake along the graft (**Figure 9**) [41, 42].

2.3 Sarcoidosis

Sarcoidosis is a multisystemic disease that most often affects the lungs and intrathoracic lymph nodes but can involve any organ in the body. The diagnosis is based on a combination of history, physical examination, radiologic and pathologic findings, and exclusion of other causes [43, 44].

^{18}F-FDG, the molecular imaging study of choice for sarcoid, with an overall sensitivity of 89–100% is more sensitive than the ACE and soluble interleukin-2 receptor tests (**Figure 10**). Whole-body imaging facilitates identification of unsuspected disease sites and guides management in these patients [45, 46]. ^{18}F-FDG is useful for monitoring treatment response. A decrease in ^{18}F-FDG lesion avidity after the initiating treatment correlates with clinical improvement, while persistent activity identifies nonresponders [47, 48].

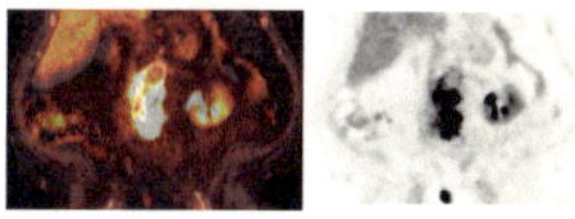

Figure 8.
Infected aortic endovascular stent. There is intense heterogeneous ^{18}F-FDG uptake surrounding the vascular stent.

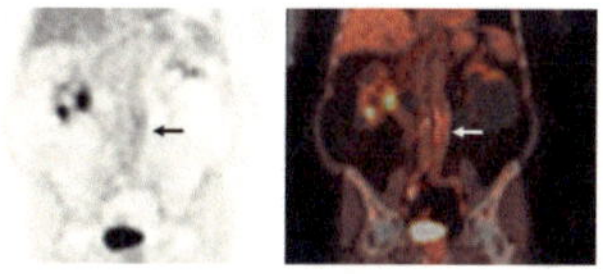

Figure 9.
Uninfected endovascular stent. There is faint homogeneous ^{18}F-FDG uptake around this stent (arrows). Compare this pattern with that of the infected stent in **Figure 8**.

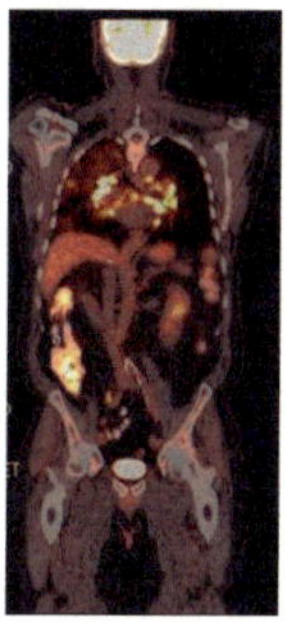

Figure 10.
Sarcoidosis. There is intense ^{18}F-FDG uptake in multiple mediastinal lymph nodes, with patchy less intense uptake in both lungs, greater on the right.

Pulmonary parenchymal uptake of ^{18}F-FDG uptake correlates with active pulmonary disease and predicts response to anti-inflammatory treatment [49]. ^{18}F-FDG uptake correlates with the bronchoalveolar lavage fluid neutrophil count and may serve as a noninvasive prognostic tool [50].

In patients with pulmonary involvement, distinguishing between fibrosis and fibrosis with active inflammation is important because patients with active inflammation could benefit from a change in therapy. Published data suggest that ^{18}F-FDG can facilitate the differentiation between pure fibrosis and fibrosis plus inflammation because pulmonary fibrotic changes do not demonstrate uptake while active lesions do. It is superior to high-resolution CT and serological evaluation for this purpose [50, 51].

2.4 Tuberculosis

Tuberculosis is the leading cause of infectious disease–related mortality worldwide. One-fourth of the world's population is latently infected and 3–5% of these individuals develop active tuberculosis disease during their lifetime. The lungs are the most common site of involvement and pulmonary disease is present in more than 80% of cases. The most common sites of extrapulmonary disease are thoracic and cervical lymph nodes, spine, adrenal glands, meninges, and gastrointestinal and genitourinary tracts [52, 53]. Early, accurate diagnosis with prompt initiation of treatment is important to minimize morbidity and mortality and to reduce the likelihood of transmission. ^{18}F-FDG is useful for identifying both pulmonary and extrapulmonary disease, measuring disease activity, identifying individuals with latent tuberculous infection at risk of developing an active infection, and monitoring response to treatment. In patients with active infection, there are two general patterns of ^{18}F-FDG uptake. The lung pattern is associated with pulmonary tuberculosis. Mediastinal lymph nodes can be slightly enlarged and demonstrate moderate ^{18}F-FDG uptake. The lymphatic pattern is associated with predominantly systemic, extra-thoracic disease. Mediastinal lymph nodes are larger and have higher ^{18}F-FDG uptake than those in patients with the lung pattern. Immunocompetent patients tend to develop the lung pattern, while immunocompromised patients are more likely to develop the lymphatic pattern [54].

Lesion activity as measured by SUV correlates with disease activity. Using dual time-point imaging, it may be possible to distinguish active from inactive pulmonary tuberculomas. Active pulmonary tuberculomas have a higher SUV max at 1 and 2 hours and a greater increase in SUV max from early to late imaging compared to inactive tuberculomas [55]. ^{18}F-FDG uptake can be present in clinically cured patients who do not go on to develop active disease. This may represent a post-treatment equilibrium in which the immune system prevents replicating bacilli from progressing to overt disease [56].

Identifying individuals with latent tuberculosis infection who are at risk of progressing to active infection is important because they should be treated. In one investigation, ^{18}F-FDG showed infiltrates and/or fibrotic scars or active nodules in ten asymptomatic subjects with an initial negative screen for active disease. These subjects were significantly more likely to have ^{18}F-FDG uptake within mediastinal lymph nodes compared to 25 subjects with either normal lung parenchyma or discrete small nodules [57].

^{18}F-FDG can assess early treatment response when radiological features may remain unchanged, with consequent significant impact on patient management. In 28 subjects with multidrug-resistant disease, ^{18}F-FDG-PET/CT performed 2 months into treatment was the best method for early prediction of treatment results and long-term outcomes [58].

In summary, ^{18}F-FDG is valuable for staging tuberculosis, locating extrapulmonary disease, identifying patients with subclinical tuberculosis, and assessing early treatment response.

2.5 Fever of unknown origin

Fever, or pyrexia, of unknown origin (FUO) is a fever that exceeds 38.3°C (101°F) on several occasions, with more than 3 weeks' duration of illness, and a failure to obtain a diagnosis after an appropriate inpatient or outpatient workup. FUO is divided into four categories: classic (the most common), nosocomial, neutropenic, and HIV-associated. Causes of classic FUO are divided into five categories: infection, neoplasm, inflammation, miscellaneous, and undiagnosed. The relative frequencies of these categories vary with the historical period, geographic region, care setting (tertiary versus community), and patient population. The etiology of FUO is undiagnosed in up to 50% of patients [59].

The workup of a patient with FUO consists of several first-line investigations: history and physical examination, laboratory tests, chest x-ray, and echocardiography when endocarditis is suspected. When first-line investigations do not yield a diagnosis, second-line procedures, including CT, MRI, and molecular imaging studies, are performed. ^{67}Ga and labeled leukocyte scintigraphy, at one time the mainstays of molecular imaging for FUO, have been replaced by ^{18}F-FDG as the molecular imaging test of choice in this population (**Figure 11**). Abnormalities identified with ^{18}F-FDG guide additional investigations that may yield a final diagnosis. A negative study excludes these conditions with a reasonable certainty, thereby avoiding unnecessary additional testing. A negative result is a good predictor of a favorable prognosis. Performed within the first 1–2 weeks in the FUO workup, ^{18}F-FDG is cost-effective by obtaining a diagnosis sooner, reducing the number of expensive, potentially invasive, diagnostic procedures performed, and decreasing the number of patients without a final diagnosis [59].

^{18}F-FDG contributes useful information in children with FUO. In one investigation, 19 (43%) of 44 scans were helpful by allowing focused evaluation in 9 cases and eliminating further workup in 10 cases [60]. In one of the largest pediatric studies to date, (n = 110) ^{18}F-FDG PET/CT established a definite diagnosis in 62% and led to treatment modification in 53% [61]. ^{18}F-FDG is helpful in children with terminal chronic liver failure and FUO during the pretransplantation period, as well as in immunocompromised children with fever [62, 63].

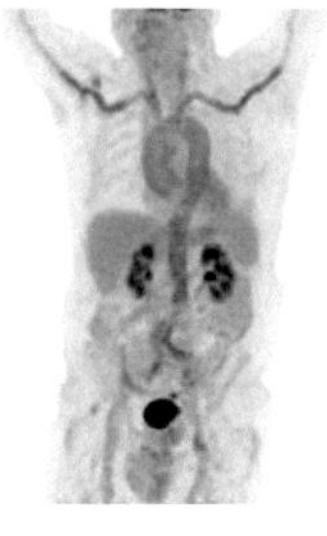

Figure 11.
Vasculitis. There is diffuse ^{18}F-FDG throughout the wall of the thoracic and abdominal aorta with extension into the subclavian and iliac arteries. ^{18}F-FDG is very sensitive for detecting large vessel vasculitis, which is a well-recognized cause of fever of unknown origin.

3. Gallium-68 citrate

For nearly 50 years, ^{67}Ga has been used for imaging infection. Now that gallium-68 citrate (^{68}Ga) is available, investigators have studied the role of this agent in diagnosing infection [64]. In a pilot study, ^{68}Ga accumulated in pulmonary and extra-pulmonary sites of disease in patients with tuberculosis was superior to CT for detecting extra-pulmonary disease. Not all pulmonary lesions concentrated ^{68}Ga and the authors hypothesized that this radiopharmaceutical might be useful for differentiating active from inactive disease and for monitoring treatment response [65]. In another investigation of patients with tuberculosis, although more lesions overall were detected with ^{18}F-FDG, brain lesions were better defined with ^{68}Ga, presumably due to the lack of physiological brain uptake of this radiopharmaceutical [66].

The potential of ^{68}Ga for diagnosing musculoskeletal infection also has been studied. In one investigation of 31 patients with suspected musculoskeletal infection, all 23 infections were detected. There were four false positive results all of which were due to tumor. Sensitivity, specificity, and accuracy were 100%, 76%, and 90%, respectively [67]. In a prospective investigation, 34 patients with clinically proven or suspected lower extremity PJI underwent ^{18}F-FDG and ^{68}Ga-citrate PET/CT. Sensitivity, specificity, and accuracy of ^{68}Ga-citrate PET/CT and ^{18}F-FDG PET/CT were 92%, 88%, and 91% and 100%, 38%, and 85%, respectively. The authors concluded that preliminary evidence suggests that ^{68}Ga-citrate PET/CT potentially could be complementary to ^{18}F-FDG PET/CT by facilitating the differentiation between infection and aseptic inflammation [68].

4. Labeled leukocytes

Although ^{18}F-FDG and ^{68}Ga are useful in the diagnostic workup of patients with infectious diseases, they are not specific and accumulate in noninfectious conditions, including benign and malignant neoplasms, and various noninfectious inflammatory conditions. Considerable effort has been devoted to developing positron-emitting radiopharmaceuticals that are specific, or at least more specific for infection, than ^{18}F-FDG and ^{68}Ga.

4.1 ^{18}F-FDG labeled leukocytes

One of the earliest attempts at creating a more specific PET radiopharmaceutical for infection imaging was the development of an *in vitro* method for labeling autologous leukocytes with ^{18}F-FDG [69, 70]. A recent meta-analysis indicates that ^{18}F-FDG labeled leukocyte imaging accurately diagnoses infection [71]. Seven studies (n = 236) were included in the meta-analysis. Pooled sensitivity was 86.3% (95%CI: 75–92.9%) and pooled specificity was 92% (95% CI: 79.8–97.1%). The positive likelihood ratio was 6.6 (95% CI: 3.1–14.1) and the negative likelihood ratio was 0.2 (95% CI: 0.12–0.33).

In spite of these favorable results, ^{18}F-FDG WBC has not been integrated into the routine diagnostic workup of infection. There are several reasons for this. Labeling efficiency is variable both in patients and normal volunteers, ranging from less than 25% to more than 95% [72–78]. This inconsistency makes it difficult to determine the quantity of ^{18}F-FDG needed for labeling leukocytes. If a worst-case labeling efficiency scenario is assumed, that is, 35%, what happens if the labeling efficiency is 80%? Is the amount of activity reinfused is reduced accordingly? If so, will the number of labeled leukocytes reinfused be adequate to provide diagnostically useful data?

Stability of the ^{18}F-FDG WBC label is another issue. In one investigation, leukocyte retention of ^{18}F-FDG decreased from 39% to 44% at 90 minutes to 19% at 4 hours [75]. In an investigation of normal volunteers, mean leukocyte retention of ^{18}F-FDG was 85% ± 4% at 1 hour, and 68% ± 7% at 4 hours [77]. In view of the degree of ^{18}F-FDG elution, one has to question whether imaging findings reflect accumulation of ^{18}F-FDG WBC, ^{18}F-FDG, or a combination.

The 110 minute physical half-life of fluorine-18 is a significant disadvantage. The time needed for *in vitro* labeling, up to 3 hours, needs to be accounted for when determining the amount of activity used to label the leukocytes. The short half-life makes it impractical for labeling to be performed off-site, which is a significant limitation in the United States where the vast majority of these labelings are performed at outside radiopharmacies. In indolent, low-grade, infections, leukocyte accumulation is slow, and imaging at later time points (e.g., 24 hours) may be necessary. The short half-life of fluorine-18 precludes imaging more than 4–5 hours after reinfusion of labeled cells. For all of these reasons, it is unlikely that ^{18}F-FDG-labeled leukocyte imaging will ever become part of mainstream clinical nuclear medicine.

4.2 Copper-64 labeled leukocytes

^{64}Cu labeling of leukocytes also has been investigated. In 10 normal volunteers, the labeling efficiency, cell viability, and stability of ^{64}Cu labeled leukocytes were compared with those of ^{111}In labeled leukocytes and ^{18}F-FDG labeled leukocytes [77]. The mean labeling efficiency for ^{64}Cu labeled leukocytes, 87% ± 4%, was nearly identical to that of ^{111}In labeled leukocytes 86% ± 4%. Leukocyte viability was the same for both radiolabels at 1 hour, 99% ± 1%, but was significantly higher for ^{64}Cu labeled leukocytes than for ^{111}In labeled leukocytes at 3 hours (98% vs. 96%, respectively) and at 24 hours (61% vs. 48%, respectively). Label stability was significantly higher for ^{111}In labeled leukocytes at 1, 2, 3, 4, and 24 hours (94%, 93%, 92%, 91%, and 88%, respectively) than for ^{64}Cu labeled leukocytes (91%, 89%, 88%, 86%, and 79%) and ^{18}F-FDG WBC (85% ± 4%, 81% ± 4%,76% ± 4%, and 68% ± 7%). Unfortunately, the labeling procedure required the use of two chelating agents: tropolone to allow the ^{64}Cu ion to enter the cell, and quin-MF/AM, to prevent elution. This complex, time-consuming procedure, which requires skilled personnel, is not well suited to routine clinical use.

Chitosan nanoparticles also have been used to label human leukocytes with ^{64}Cu. The labeling efficiency was only about 26% and more than 90% of the activity had eluted from the leukocytes at 2 hours [79].

4.3 Zirconium-89 labeled leukocytes

^{89}Zr, with a half-life of 78.4 hours, has also been used to label leukocytes *in vitro*. In one investigation, chitosan nanoparticles were used to label human leukocytes with ^{89}Zr. Labeling efficiency was 76.8%. Cell viability at the completion of labeling was 61%; 28.4% of the intracellular activity had eluted at 2 hours, 35.2% at 4 hours, and 53.3% at 24 hours. The entire labeling process took nearly 6 hours to complete. In this investigation, only 61% of the labeled leukocytes were viable.

Recent investigations are more promising. In one study, *in vitro* labeling of human leukocytes with ^{89}Zr-oxine was compared to labeling with ^{111}In-oxine [80]. Labeling efficiency for ^{89}Zr labeled leukocytes was 48.7% vs. 89.1% ($P < 0.0001$) for ^{111}In labeled leukocytes. However, there were no significant differences between ^{89}Zr labeled leukocytes and ^{111}In labeled leukocytes with respect to elution of activity or cell viability. Another group obtained similar results when using ^{89}Zr-oxinate4 to label human leukocytes [81]. These results are encouraging, but *in vivo* investigations of ^{89}Zr labeled leukocytes to diagnose infection are lacking.

5. Infection-specific agents

5.1 Iodine-124 fialuridine

The radioiodinated thymidine analog fialuridine (FIAU) was developed for reporter genes, for cells that were transfected with herpes simplex virus thymidine kinase (TK). This enzyme transfers a phosphate group from ATP to pyrimidine deoxynucleoside. The lipophilic agent diffuses into the cell where it is trapped with the TK activity [82]. FIAU is also phosphorylated by endogenous bacterial TK. In a pilot investigation, ^{124}I-FIAU PET/CT successfully detected musculoskeletal infection in seven patients and was negative in one healthy control [83]. Results of subsequent investigations of ^{124}I-FIAU for diagnosing musculoskeletal infection were less satisfactory. In 19 subjects with suspected lower extremity PJI, image quality was suboptimal because of metal artifact and high nonspecific muscle uptake [84]. In an investigation of ^{124}I FIAU for diagnosing foot osteomyelitis in diabetics the study was terminated because of a lack of correlation between ^{124}I FIAU uptake and bone biopsy results [85].

5.2 Fluorine-18 fluorodeoxysorbitol

Sorbitol, a sugar alcohol, is a metabolic substrate for Enterobacteriaceae, the largest group of Gram-negative bacterial pathogens in humans. Sorbitol is selectively taken up by bacteria *via* surface transporters, phosphorylated, and further metabolized [86]. The radiolabeled sorbitol analog, ^{18}F-FDS rapidly and selectively accumulates in Enterobacteriaceae. In a murine myositis model, ^{18}F-FDS PET rapidly differentiated infection from sterile inflammation [87]. ^{18}F-FDS was determined to be safe and well tolerated after a single intravenous dose was injected into healthy human volunteers to assess biodistribution and radiation dosimetry [88].

In a prospective investigation of 26 patients, ^{18}F-FDS PET/CT was safe, rapidly localized Enterobacterales infections and differentiated them from sterile inflammation and tumor. Follow-up imaging in the same patients performed for monitoring antibiotic treatment demonstrated decreased uptake correlating with clinical improvement [89].

5.3 Antimicrobial peptides

Antimicrobial peptides (AMPs) bind to the bacterial cell membrane. Their expression may be constant or induced by contact with microbes. They also may be transported to sites of infection by leukocytes [90]. Radiolabeled synthetic fragments of ubiquicidin, a naturally occurring human AMP that targets bacteria, possess the ability to differentiate infection from sterile inflammation and have shown potential for monitoring treatment in staphylococcus aureus infections [91–93].

Although ^{99m}Tc labeled AMPS have been used in most investigations, preclinical data indicate that ^{68}Ga labeled AMPS can be used to detect and localize infection [94]. ^{68}Ga-DOTA-TBIA101 successfully detected *E. coli*-infected muscle tissue in mice. Normalization of the infected thigh muscle to reference tissue showed a ratio of 3.0 ± 0.8 and a ratio of 2.3 ± 0.6 compared to the identical healthy [95]. Although these results are encouraging, at the present time human data are too few to draw any conclusions about the clinical utility of these agents.

6. Conclusions

^{18}F-FDG is extremely useful in the diagnostic workup of patients suspected of having infection. It has emerged as the molecular imaging test of choice for spondylodiscitis, FUO in both adults and children, sarcoid, and vasculitis. This test is also valuable in the diagnostic workup of patients with diabetic foot and cardiovascular infections. The most significant limitation of ^{18}F-FDG is a lack of specificity. Investigators have sought to capitalize on the advantages of PET over single photon emitting radiopharmaceuticals, by developing PET radiopharmaceuticals that are more specific for infection. Early efforts focused on *in vitro* labeling of leukocytes with PET radiopharmaceuticals but for a variety of reasons, these agents have not entered the clinical arena, nor is it likely that they will. Initial results with ^{124}I-FIAU were encouraging, but subsequent data dampened the enthusiasm for this agent. Based on preliminary data, ^{18}F-FDS and ^{68}Ga labeled siderophores and AMPs show promise as infection-specific agents. However, clinical trials are needed to establish their value.

Conflict of interest

The author declares no conflict of interest.

Author details

Christopher J. Palestro
Donald and Barbara Zucker School of Medicine at Hofstra/Northwell, New York, USA

*Address all correspondence to: palestro@northwell.edu

IntechOpen

© 2023 The Author(s). Licensee IntechOpen. This chapter is distributed under the terms of the Creative Commons Attribution License (http://creativecommons.org/licenses/by/3.0), which permits unrestricted use, distribution, and reproduction in any medium, provided the original work is properly cited. (cc) BY

References

[1] Palestro CJ. Molecular imaging of infection: the first 50 years. Seminars in Nuclear Medicine. 2020;**50**:23-34. DOI: 10.1053/j.semnuclmed.2019.10.002

[2] Zhuang H, Alavi A. 18-fluorodeoxyglucose positron emission tomographic imaging in the detection and monitoring of infection and inflammation. Seminars in Nuclear Medicine. 2002;**32**:47-59. DOI: 10.1053/snuc.2002.29278

[3] Meller J, Sahlmann CO, Scheel AK. 18F-FDG PET and PET/CT in fever of unknown origin. Journal of Nuclear Medicine. 2007;**48**:35-45

[4] Love C, Tomas MB, Tronco GG, Palestro CJ. FDG PET of infection and inflammation. Radiographics. 2005;**25**:1357-1368. DOI: 10.1148/rg.255045122

[5] Palestro CJ. FDG PET in musculoskeletal infection. Seminars in Nuclear Medicine. 2013;**43**:367-376. DOI: 10.1053/j.semnuclmed.2013.04.006

[6] Wang GL, Zhao K, Liu ZF, Dong MJ, Yang SY. A meta-analysis of fluorodeoxyglucose-positron emission tomography versus scintigraphy in the evaluation of suspected osteomyelitis. Nuclear Medicine Communications. 2011;**32**:1134-1142. DOI: 10.1097/MNM.0b013e32834b455c

[7] Termaat MF, Raijmakers PG, Scholten HJ, et al. The accuracy of diagnostic imaging for the assessment of chronic osteomyelitis: a systematic review and meta-analysis. The Journal of Bone and Joint Surgery. American Volume. 2005;**87**:2464-2471. DOI: 10.2106/JBJS.D.02691

[8] Prodromou ML, Ziakas PD, Poulou LS, Karsaliakos P, Thanos L, Mylonakis E. FDG PET is a robust tool for the diagnosis of spondylodiscitis: a meta-analysis of diagnostic data. Clinical Nuclear Medicine. 2014;**39**:330-335. DOI: 10.1097/RLU.0000000000000336

[9] Treglia G, Pascale M, Lazzeri E, van der Bruggen W, Delgado Bolton RC, Glaudemans AWJM. Diagnostic performance of 18F-FDG PET/CT in patients with spinal infection: a systematic review and a bivariate meta-analysis. European Journal of Nuclear Medicine and Molecular Imaging. 2020;**47**:1287-1301. DOI: 10.1007/s00259-019-04571-6

[10] Gratz S, Dorner J, Fischer U, et al. 18F-FDG hybrid PET in patients with suspected spondylitis. European Journal of Nuclear Medicine and Molecular Imaging. 2002;**29**:516-524

[11] Fuster D, Solà O, Soriano A, et al. A prospective study comparing whole-body FDG PET/CT to combined planar bone scan with 67Ga SPECT/CT in the diagnosis of spondylodiskitis. Clinical Nuclear Medicine. 2012;**37**:827-832. DOI: 10.1097/RLU.0b013e318262ae6c

[12] Frenkel Rutenberg T, Baruch Y, Ohana N, et al. The role of 18F-fluorodeoxyglucose positron-emission tomography/computed tomography in the diagnosis of postoperative hardware-related spinal Infections. The Israel Medical Association Journal. 2019;**21**(8):532-537

[13] Skanjeti A, Penna D, Douroukas A, et al. PET in the clinical work-up of patients with spondylodiscitis: a new tool for the clinician? The Quarterly Journal

of Nuclear Medicine and Molecular Imaging. 2012;**56**:569-576

[14] Kim SJ, Kim IJ, Suh KT, et al. Prediction of residual disease of spine infection using F-18 FDG PET/CT. Spine. 2009;**34**:2424-2430. DOI: 10.1097/BRS.0b013e3181b1fd33

[15] Nanni C, Boriani L, Salvadori C, et al. FDG PET/CT is useful for the interim evaluation of response to therapy in patients affected by haematogenous spondylodiscitis. European Journal of Nuclear Medicine and Molecular Imaging. 2012;**39**:1538-1544. DOI: 10.1007/s00259-012-2179-8

[16] Ioannou S, Chatziioannou S, Pneumaticos SG, Zormpala A, Sipsas NV. Fluorine-18 fluoro-2-deoxy-D-glucose positron emission tomography/computed tomography scan contributes to the diagnosis and management of brucellar spondylodiskitis. BMC Infectious Diseases. 2013;**13**:73. DOI: 10.1186/1471-2334-13-73

[17] Righi E, Carnelutti A, Muser D, et al. Incremental value of FDG-PET/CT to monitor treatment response in infectious spondylodiscitis. Skeletal Radiology. 2020;**49**:903-912. DOI: 10.1007/s00256-019-03328-4

[18] Riccio SA, Chu AK, Rabin HR, Kloiber R. Fluorodeoxyglucose positron emission tomography/computed tomography interpretation criteria for assessment of antibiotic treatment response in pyogenic spine infection. Canadian Association of Radiologists Journal. 2015;**66**:145-152. DOI: 10.1016/j.carj.2014.08.004

[19] Yu GJ, Koslowsky IL, Riccio SA, Chu AKM, Rabin HR, Kloiber R. Diagnostic challenges in pyogenic spinal infection: an expanded role for FDG-PET/CT. European Journal of Clinical Microbiology & Infectious Diseases. 2018;**37**:501-509. DOI: 10.1007/s10096-018-3197-7

[20] Palestro CJ, Love C. Nuclear medicine and diabetic foot infections. Seminars in Nuclear Medicine. 2009;**39**:52-65. DOI: 10.1053/j.semnuclmed.2008.08.006

[21] Treglia G, Sadeghi R, Annunziata S, et al. Diagnostic performance of fluorine-18-fluorodeoxyglucose positron emission tomography for the diagnosis of osteomyelitis related to diabetic foot: a systematic review and a meta-analysis. Foot (Edinburgh, Scotland). 2013;**23**:140-148. DOI: 10.1016/j.foot.2013.07.002

[22] Lauri C, Tamminga M, Glaudemans AWJM, et al. Detection of osteomyelitis in the diabetic foot by imaging techniques: a systematic review and meta-analysis comparing MRI, white blood cell scintigraphy, and FDG-PET. Diabetes Care. 2017;**40**:1111-1120. DOI: 10.2337/dc17-0532

[23] Jin H, Yuan L, Li C, Kan Y, Hao R, Yang J. Diagnostic performance of FDG PET or PET/CT in prosthetic infection after arthroplasty: a meta-analysis. The Quarterly Journal of Nuclear Medicine and Molecular Imaging. 2014;**58**:85-93

[24] Kwee TC, Kwee RM, Alavi A. FDG-PET for diagnosing prosthetic joint infection: Systematic review and metaanalysis. European Journal of Nuclear Medicine and Molecular Imaging. 2008;**35**:2122-2132. DOI: 10.1007/s00259-008-0887-x

[25] Palestro CJ. Molecular Imaging of Periprosthetic Joint Infections. Seminars in Nuclear Medicine. 2023;**52**:167-174. DOI: 10.1053/j.semnuclmed.2022.11.004

[26] Pinski JM, Chen AF, Estok DM, Kavolus JJ. Nuclear medicine scans in

total joint replacement. Journal of Bone and Joint Surgery. 2011;**103**:359-372. DOI: 10.2106/JBJS.20.00301

[27] Falstie-Jensen T, Lange J, Daugaard H, et al. 18F FDG-PET/CT has poor diagnostic accuracy in diagnosing shoulder PJI. European Journal of Nuclear Medicine and Molecular Imaging. 2019;**46**:2013-2022. DOI: 10.1007/s00259-019-04381-w

[28] Holland TL, Baddour LM, Bayer AS, Hoen B, Miro JM, Fowler VG Jr. Infective endocarditis. Nature Reviews. Disease Primers. 2016;**2**:16059. DOI: 10.1038/nrdp.2016.59

[29] Erba PA, Conti U, Lazzeri E, et al. Added value of 99mTc-HMPAO-labeled leukocyte SPECT/CT in the characterization and management of patients with infectious endocarditis. Journal of Nuclear Medicine. 2012;**53**:1235-1243. DOI: 10.2967/jnumed.111.099424

[30] Yan J, Zhang C, Niu Y, et al. The role of 18F-FDG PET/CT in infectious endocarditis: a systematic review and meta-analysis. International Journal of Clinical Pharmacology and Therapeutics. 2016;**54**:337-342. DOI: 10.5414/CP202569

[31] Rouzet F, Chequer R, Benali K, et al. Respective performance of 18F-FDG PET and radiolabeled leukocyte scintigraphy for the diagnosis of prosthetic valve endocarditis. Journal of Nuclear Medicine. 2014;**55**:1980-1985. DOI: 10.2967/jnumed.114.141895

[32] Baddour LM, Epstein AE, Erickson CC, et al. Update on cardiovascular implantable electronic device infections and their management: a scientific statement from the American Heart Association. Circulation. 2010;**121**:458-477. DOI: 10.1161/CIRCULATIONAHA.109.192665

[33] Pizzi MN, Roque A, Fernández-Hidalgo N, et al. Improving the diagnosis of infective endocarditis in prosthetic valves and intracardiac devices with 18F-Fluordeoxyglucose positron emission tomography/computed tomography angiography: initial results at an infective endocarditis referral center. Circulation. 2015;**132**:1113-1126. DOI: 10.1161/CIRCULATIONAHA.115.015316

[34] Bensimhon L, Lavergne T, Hugonnet F, et al. Whole body [(18) F] fluorodeoxyglucose positron emission tomography imaging for the diagnosis of pacemaker or implantable cardioverter defibrillator infection: a preliminary prospective study. Clinical Microbiology and Infection. 2011;**17**:836-844. DOI: 10.1111/j.1469-0691.2010.03312.x

[35] Sarrazin JF, Philippon F, Tessier M, et al. Usefulness of fluorine-18 positron emission tomography/computed tomography for identification of cardiovascular implantable electronic device infections. Journal of the American College of Cardiology. 2012;**59**:1616-1625. DOI: 10.1016/j.jacc.2011.11.059

[36] Dell'Aquila AM, Mastrobuoni S, Alles S, et al. Contributory role of fluorine 18-fluorodeoxyglucose positron emission tomography/computed tomography in the diagnosis and clinical management of infections in patients supported with a continuous-flow left ventricular assist device. The Annals of Thoracic Surgery. 2016;**101**:87-94. DOI: 10.1016/j.athoracsur.2015.06.066

[37] Mahmood M, Kendi AT, Farid S, et al. Role of 18F-FDG PET/CT in the diagnosis of cardiovascular implantable electronic device infections: a meta-analysis. Journal of Nuclear Cardiology. 2019;**26**:958-970. DOI: 10.1007/s12350-017-1063-0

[38] Wilson WR, Bower TC, Creager MA, et al. Vascular graft infections, mycotic aneurysms, and endovascular infections: a scientific statement from the American Heart Association. Circulation. 2016;**134**:e412-e460. DOI: 10.1161/CIR.0000000000000457

[39] Keidar Z, Engel A, Hoffman A, Israel O, Nitecki S. Prosthetic vascular graft infection: the role of 18F-FDG PET/CT. Journal of Nuclear Medicine. 2007;**48**:1230-1126. DOI: 10.2967/jnumed.107.040253

[40] Sah BR, Husmann L, Mayer D, et al. VASGRA Cohort. Diagnostic performance of 18F-FDG-PET/CT in vascular graft infections. European Journal of Vascular and Endovascular Surgery. 2015;**49**:455-464. DOI: 10.1016/j.ejvs.2014.12.024

[41] Keidar Z, Pirmisashvili N, Leiderman M, Nitecki S, Israel O. 18F-FDG uptake in noninfected prosthetic vascular grafts: incidence, patterns, and changes over time. Journal of Nuclear Medicine. 2014;**55**:392-395. DOI: 10.2967/jnumed.113.128173

[42] Saleem BR, Pol RA, Slart RH, Reijnen MM, Zeebregts CJ. 18F-Fluorodeoxyglucose positron emission tomography/CT scanning in diagnosing vascular prosthetic graft infection. BioMed Research International. 2014;**2014**:471971. DOI: 10.1155/2014/471971

[43] Llanos O, Hamzeh N. Sarcoidosis. The Medical Clinics of North America. 2019;**103**:527-534. DOI: 10.1016/j.mcna.2018.12.011

[44] Brown F, Modi P, Tanner LS. Lofgren syndrome. 2020 Aug 8. In: StatPearls. StatPearls Publishing; 2022. Bookshelf ID: NBK482315

[45] Keijsers RGM, Grutters JC. In which patients with sarcoidosis is FDG PET/CT indicated? Journal of Clinical Medicine. 2020;**9**:890. DOI: 10.3390/jcm9030890

[46] Akaike G, Itani M, Shah H, et al. PET/CT in the diagnosis and workup of sarcoidosis: focus on atypical manifestations. Radiographics. 2018;**38**:1536-1549. DOI: 10.1148/rg.2018180053

[47] Sobic-Saranovic D, Grozdic I, Videnovic-Ivanov J, et al. The utility of 18F-FDG PET/CT for diagnosis and adjustment of therapy in patients with active chronic sarcoidosis. Journal of Nuclear Medicine. 2012;**53**:1543-1549. DOI: 10.2967/jnumed.112.104380

[48] Maturu VN, Rayamajhi SJ, Agarwal R, Aggarwal AN, Gupta D, Mittal BR. Role of serial F-18 FDG PET/CT scans in assessing treatment response and predicting relapses in patients with symptomatic sarcoidosis. Sarcoidosis, Vasculitis, and Diffuse Lung Diseases. 2016;**33**:372-380

[49] Keijsers RG, Verzijlbergen JF, van Diepen DM, van den Bosch JM, Grutters JC. 18F-FDG PET in sarcoidosis: an observational study in 12 patients treated with infliximab. Sarcoidosis, Vasculitis, and Diffuse Lung Diseases. 2008;**25**:143-149

[50] Guleria R, Jyothidasan A, Madan K, et al. Utility of FDG-PET-CT scanning in assessing the extent of disease activity and response to treatment in sarcoidosis. Lung India. 2014;**31**:323-330. DOI: 10.4103/0970-2113.142092

[51] Mostard RL, Vöö S, van Kroonenburgh MJ, et al. Inflammatory activity assessment by F18 FDG-PET/CT in persistent symptomatic sarcoidosis. Respiratory Medicine. 2011;**105**:1917-1924. DOI: 10.1016/j.rmed.2011.08.012

[52] Yu WY, Lu PX, Assadi M, et al. Updates on 18F-FDG-PET/CT as a clinical tool for tuberculosis evaluation and therapeutic monitoring. Quantitative Imaging in Medicine and Surgery. 2019;**9**:1132-1146. DOI: 10.21037/qims.2019.05.24

[53] Ankrah AO, Glaudemans AWJM, Maes A, et al. Tuberculosis. Seminars in Nuclear Medicine. 2018;**48**:108-130. DOI: 10.1053/j.semnuclmed.2017.10.005

[54] Soussan M, Brillet PY, Mekinian A, et al. Patterns of pulmonary tuberculosis on FDG-PET/CT. European Journal of Radiology. 2012;**81**:2872-2286. DOI: 10.1016/j.ejrad.2011.09.002

[55] Kim IJ, Lee JS, Kim SJ, et al. Double-phase 18F-FDG PET-CT for determination of pulmonary tuberculoma activity. European Journal of Nuclear Medicine and Molecular Imaging. 2008;**35**:808-814. DOI: 10.1007/s00259-007-0585-0

[56] Malherbe ST, Shenai S, Ronacher K, et al. Persisting positron emission tomography lesion activity and Mycobacterium tuberculosis mRNA after tuberculosis cure. Nature Medicine. 2016;**22**:1094-1100. DOI: 10.1038/nm.4177

[57] Esmail H, Lai RP, Lesosky M, et al. Characterization of progressive HIV-associated tuberculosis using 2-deoxy-2-[18F]fluoro-D-glucose positron emission and computed tomography. Nature Medicine. 2016;**22**:1090-1093. DOI: 10.1038/nm.4161

[58] Chen RY, Dodd LE, Lee M, et al. PET/CT imaging correlates with treatment outcome in patients with multidrug-resistant tuberculosis. Science Translational Medicine. 2014;**6**:265ra166. DOI: 10.1126/scitranslmed.3009501

[59] Palestro CJ, Brandon D, Dibble EH, Keidar Z, Kwak J. FDG PET in evaluation of patients with fever of unknown origin: AJR Expert Panel Narrative Review. AJR. American Journal of Roentgenology. DOI: 10.2214/AJR.22.28726 [Online ahead of print]

[60] Jasper N, Dabritz J, Frosch M, Loeffler M, Weckesser M, Foell D. Diagnostic value of 18F-FDG PET/CT in children with fever of unknown origin or unexplained signs of inflammation. European Journal of Nuclear Medicine and Molecular Imaging. 2010;**37**:136-145. DOI: 10.1007/s00259-009-1185-y

[61] Pijl JP, Kwee TC, Legger GE, et al. Role of FDG-PET/CT in children with fever of unknown origin. European Journal of Nuclear Medicine and Molecular Imaging. 2020;**47**:1596-1604. DOI: 10.1007/s00259-020-04707-z

[62] Sturm E, Rings EH, Scholvinck EH, Gouw AS, Porte RJ, Pruim J. Fluordeoxyglucose positron emission tomography contributes to management of pediatric liver transplantation candidates with fever of unknown origin. Liver Transplantation. 2006;**12**:1698-1704. DOI: 10.1002/lt.20922

[63] Wang SS, Mechinaud F, Thursky K, Cain T, Lau E, Haeusler GM. The clinical utility of fluorodeoxyglucose positron emission tomography for investigation of fever in immunocompromised children. Journal of Paediatrics and Child Health. 2018;**54**:487-492. DOI: doi.org/10.1111/jpc.13809

[64] Kumar V, Boddeti DK, Evans SG, Angelides S. 68Ga-citrate-PET for diagnostic imaging of infection in rats and for intra-abdominal infection in a patient. Current Radiopharmaceuticals. 2012;**5**:71-75. DOI: 10.2174/1874471011205010071

[65] Vorster M, Maes A, Van de Wiele C, Sathekge MM. 68Ga-citrate PET/CT in tuberculosis: a pilot study. The Quarterly

Journal of Nuclear Medicine and Molecular Imaging. 2019;**63**:48-55. DOI: 10.23736/S1824-4785.16.02680-7

[66] Ankrah AO, Lawal IO, Boshomane TMG, et al. Comparison of Fluorine(18)-fluorodeoxyglucose and Gallium(68)-citrate PET/CT in patients with tuberculosis. Nuklearmedizin. 2019;**58**:371-378. DOI: 10.1055/a-1000-6951

[67] Nanni C, Errani C, Boriani L, et al. 68Ga-Citrate PET/CT for evaluating patients with infections of the bone: preliminary results. Journal of Nuclear Medicine. 2010;**51**:1932-1936. DOI: 10.2967/jnumed.110.080184

[68] Tseng JR, Chang YH, Yang LY, et al. Potential usefulness of 68Ga-citrate PET/CT in detecting infected lower limb prostheses. EJNMMI Research. 2019;**9**(1):2. DOI: 10.1186/s13550-018-0468-3

[69] Forstrom LA, Mullan BP, Hung JC, Lowe VJ, Thorson LM. 18F-FDG labelling of human leukocytes. Nuclear Medicine Communications. 2000;**21**:691-694. DOI:10.1097/00006231-200007000-00014

[70] Forstrom LA, Dunn WL, Mullan BP, Hung JC, Lowe VJ, Thorson LM. Biodistribution and dosimetry of [(18)F] fluorodeoxyglucose labelled leukocytes in normal human subjects. Nuclear Medicine Communications. 2002;**23**:721-725. DOI:10.1097/00006231-200208000-00004

[71] Meyer M, Testart N, Jreige M, et al. Diagnostic performance of PET or PET/CT using 18F-FDG labeled white blood cells in infectious diseases: a systematic review and a bivariate meta-analysis. Diagnostics (Basel). 2019;**9**:60. DOI: 10.3390/diagnostics9020060

[72] Aksoy SY, Asa S, Ozhan M, et al. FDG and FDG-labelled leucocyte PET/CT in the imaging of prosthetic joint infection. European Journal of Nuclear Medicine and Molecular Imaging. 2014;**41**:556-564. DOI: 10.1007/s00259-013-2597-2

[73] Bhattacharya A, Kochhar R, Sharma S, et al. PET/CT with 18F-FDG-labeled autologous leukocytes for the diagnosis of infected fluid collections in acute pancreatitis. Journal of Nuclear Medicine. 2014;**55**:1267-1272. DOI: 10.2967/jnumed.114.137232

[74] Dumarey N, Egrise D, Blocklet D, et al. Imaging infection with 18F-FDG-labeled leukocyte PET/CT: initial experience in 21 patients. Journal of Nuclear Medicine. 2006;**47**:625-632

[75] Pellegrino D, Bonab AA, Dragotakes SC, Pitman JT, Mariani G, Carter EA. 2005. Inflammation and infection: imaging properties of 18F-FDG-labeled white blood cells versus 18F-FDG. Journal of Nuclear Medicine. 2005;**46**:1522-1530

[76] Rini JN, Bhargava KK, Tronco GG, et al. PET with FDG-labeled leukocytes versus scintigraphy with 111In-oxine-labeled leukocytes for detection of infection. Radiology. 2006;**238**:978-987. DOI: 10.1148/radiol.2382041993

[77] Bhargava KK, Gupta RK, Nichols KJ, Palestro CJ. In vitro human leukocyte labeling with (64)Cu: an intraindividual comparison with (111)In-oxine and (18)F-FDG. Nuclear Medicine and Biology. 2009;**36**:545-549. DOI: 10.1016/j.nucmedbio.2009.03.001

[78] Lafont P, Morelec I, Fraysse M, et al. 18F-FDG labelled leukocytes in vitro functional tests: viability, chemotaxis and phagocytosis assays. The Open Nuclear Medicine Journal. 2011;**3**:25-29. DOI: 10.2174/1876388X01103010025

[79] Fairclough M, Prenant C, Ellis B, et al. A new technique for the

radiolabelling of mixed leukocytes with zirconium-89 for inflammation imaging with positron emission tomography. Journal of Labelled Compounds and Radiopharmaceuticals. 2016;**59**:270-276. DOI: 10.1002/jlcr.3392

[80] Man F, Khan AA, Carrascal-Miniño A, Blower PJ, TM de Rosales R. A kit formulation for the preparation of [89Zr]Zr(oxinate)4 for PET cell tracking: white blood cell labelling and comparison with [111In]In(oxinate)3. Nuclear Medicine and Biology. 2020;**90-91**:31-40. DOI: 10.1016/j.nucmedbio.2020.09.002

[81] Massicano AVF, Bartels JL, Jeffers CD, et al. Production of [89 Zr]Oxinate4 and cell radiolabeling for human use. Journal of Labelled Compounds and Radiopharmaceuticals. 2021;**64**:209-216. DOI: 10.1002/jlcr.3901

[82] Boerman OC, Laverman P, Oyen WJ. FIAU: from reporter gene imaging to imaging of bacterial proliferation. American Journal of Nuclear Medicine and Molecular Imaging. 2012;**2**:271-272

[83] Diaz LA, Foss CA, Thornton K, et al. Imaging of musculoskeletal bacterial infections by [124I]FIAU-PET/CT. PLoS One. 2007;**10**:e1007. DOI: 10.1371/journal.pone.0001007

[84] Zhang XM, Zhang HH, McLeroth P, et al. [124I]FIAU: Human dosimetry and infection imaging in patients with suspected prosthetic joint infection. Nuclear Medicine and Biology. 2016;**43**:273-279. DOI: 10.1016/j.nucmedbio.2016.01.004

[85] [124I]FIAU-PET/CT scanning in diagnosing osteomyelitis in patients with diabetic foot. Available from: infection.clinicaltrials.gov/ct2/show/NCT01764919. Updated 6 April 2016. [Accessed: 14 February 2023]

[86] Lengeler J. Nature and properties of hexitol transport systems in Escherichia coli. Journal of Bacteriology. 1975;**124**:39-47. DOI: 10.1128/jb.124.1.39-47.1975

[87] Weinstein EA, Ordonez AA, DeMarco VP, et al. Imaging Enterobacteriaceae infection in vivo with 18F-fluorodeoxysorbitol positron emission tomography. Science Translational Medicine. 2014;**6**(259):259ra146. DOI: 10.1126/scitranslmed.3009815

[88] Zhu W, Yao S, Xing H, et al. Biodistribution and radiation dosimetry of the enterobacteriaceae-specific imaging probe [18F]Fluorodeoxysorbitol determined by PET/CT in healthy human volunteers. Molecular Imaging and Biology. 2016;**18**:782-787. DOI: 10.1007/s11307-016-0946-9

[89] Ordonez AA, Wintaco LM, Mota F, et al. Imaging Enterobacterales infections in patients using pathogen-specific positron emission tomography. Science Translational Medicine. 2021, 2021;**13**(589):eabe9805. DOI: 10.1126/scitranslmed.abe9805

[90] Lupetti A, Pauwels EKJ, Nibbering PH, Welling MM. 99mTc-antimicrobial peptides: promising candidates for infection imaging. The Quarterly Journal of Nuclear Medicine. 2003;**47**:238-245

[91] Lupetti A, Welling MM, Mazzi U, Nibbering PH, Pauwels EKJ. Technetium-99m labelled fluconazole and antimicrobial peptides for imaging of Candida albicans and Aspergillus fumigatus infections. European Journal of Nuclear Medicine and Molecular Imaging. 2002;**29**:674-679. DOI: 10.1007/s00259-001-0760-7

[92] Sarda-Mantel L, Saleh-Mghir A, Welling MM, et al. Evaluation of

99mTc-UBI 29-41 scintigraphy for specific detection of experimental Staphylococcus aureus prosthetic joint infections. European Journal of Nuclear Medicine and Molecular Imaging. 2007;**34**:1302-1309. DOI: 10.1007/s00259-007-0368-7

[93] Meléndez-Alafort L, Rodríguez-Cortés J, Ferro-Flores G, et al. Biokinetics of (99m)Tc-UBI 29-41 in humans. Nuclear Medicine and Biology. 2004;**31**:373-379. DOI: 10.1016/j.nucmedbio.2003.10.005

[94] Ebenhan T, Chadwick N, Sathekge MM, et al. Peptide synthesis, characterization and ^{68}Ga-radiolabeling of NOTA-conjugated ubiquicidin fragments for prospective infection imaging with PET/CT. Nuclear Medicine and Biology. 2014;**41**:390-400. DOI: 10.1016/j.nucmedbio.2014.02.001

[95] Mokaleng BB, Ebenhan T, Ramesh S, et al. Synthesis, 68Ga-radiolabeling, and preliminary in vivo assessment of a depsipeptide-derived compound as a potential PET/CT infection imaging agent. BioMed Research International. 2015;**2015**:284354. DOI: 10.1155/2015/284354

Section 2

Diagnosis and Management of Constructive Pericarditis

Chapter 3

Constrictive Pericarditis

Francesco Maria Lauri

Abstract

Constrictive pericarditis (CP) is a challenging clinical scenario in which the heart muscle is entrapped by thick, fibrous, and frequently calcified pericardial layers. Whereas infectious diseases (mostly bacterial) had been observed as the main etiology in the last decades, nowadays, post-surgical or radiotherapy iatrogenic inflammation is becoming highly prevalent with the exception of developing countries and patients with immunodeficiency in which tuberculosis is still frequently observed. Clinically, progressive dyspnea and peripheral edema are present and frequently considered of unknown origin because of the diagnostic challenge that CP poses. As a matter of fact, a specific knowledge of echocardiography and right heart catheterization is essential to recognize constriction features. Moreover, a valuable support is provided by dedicated imaging modalities (mostly magnetic resonance). Complete surgical removal of the pericardium (pericardiectomy), when feasible and performed early, is associated with excellent symptomatic improvement. Unfortunately, in specific scenarios (radiation therapy) or when surgery is performed after severe constriction development, surgical outcomes are poor, and CP assumes the profile of an end-stage disease. This reinforces the unmet need of early detection of CP and the development of novel therapeutic strategies.

Keywords: constrictive pericarditis, right heart catheterization, pericardiectomy, heart failure, restrictive cardiomyopathy

1. Introduction

Constrictive pericarditis (CP), firstly described by Richard Lower in "*Tractatus de Corde*" (1669), is the end-stage evolution of chronic inflammation and fibrosis of pericardium. Many of the causes of acute pericarditis listed in previous chapters have been associated with the development of pericardial constriction weeks to months after the acute episode. Nonetheless, the appearance of progressive dyspnea and peripheral edema are not promptly addressed to CP and are frequently considered of unknown origin because of the diagnostic challenge that CP poses [1]. As a matter of fact, diagnosis of CP can be challenging because of the low prevalence (<1% of acute pericarditis, 0.2–0.4% of patients submitted to cardiac surgery) and subsequent detraining of echocardiography specialists. Moreover, constrictive hemodynamics can be difficult to distinguish from restrictive cardiomyopathy (RCM) physiology, a primary myocardial disease, and finally, pericardium could present a normal thickness in almost 20% of CP cases with calcifications present in less than half of patients [2].

IntechOpen

2. Etiology

Traditionally, CP had been described months to years after acute bacterial pericarditis, whereas in the last decades, chronic inflammation associated with previous thoracic surgery or radiotherapy has become the most frequent cause of CP. A recent meta-analysis of patients submitted to pericardiectomy for symptomatic CP [2] has collected data about 2114 patients admitted between 1991 and 2019. Idiopathic etiology was present in approximately half of patients (50.2%) followed by post-cardiac surgery (26.2%) and mediastinal radiotherapy (8.9%). Interestingly, studies published after 2000 have reported a dramatic decrease of cases secondary to cardiac surgery with respect to previous reports (15% vs. 33%, $p < .001$). This could reflect the evolution of cardiac surgery techniques with progressively reduced operative times and close echocardiographic evaluation after surgery.

Moreover, end-stage renal disease, connective tissue disorders (i.e., lupus erythematosus, rheumatoid arthritis, systemic sclerosis, etc.), and pulmonary diseases, including pulmonary asbestosis and mesothelioma infiltrating the pericardium, are less frequent but important causes of CP. More exceptional is CP secondary to transmural myocardial infarction (Dressler's syndrome), given the spread of primary angioplasty and, consequently, the reduction of infarct size, in developed countries. Finally, CP secondary to tuberculosis infection in developed countries has been reported to be a rare condition (3%) with an increasing trend in the last decades due to imported cases and the spread of HIV infections. Nonetheless, taking into account socioeconomic background, tuberculosis infections and, along with them, late complications like CP are significantly increasing in developing countries. Consequently, tuberculosis has become the first cause of CP in countries of sub-Saharan Africa and few countries of Asia, including India where tuberculosis was associated with more than half of cases of CP (51.6%) in a retrospective single-center analysis, including patients submitted to pericardiectomy between 2009 and 2020 [3].

3. Pathophysiology

Chronic pericardial inflammation usually drives a structural change of pericardial layers, resulting in progressive fibrosis and calcifications and leading to partial adhesions between the layers. Consequently, difficulties in diastolic ventricle filling can be observed. As a matter of fact, during diastole, ventricles experience an active (ATP-consuming) relaxation with a rapid decrease of chamber pressures leading to mitral valve opening and early inflow with a velocity as higher as the pressure gradient between atrial and ventricular chambers. This phase is usually followed by an atrial contraction leading to further ventricle filling with no significant increase of end-diastolic ventricular pressures unless pathologic conditions, like CP, occur. In case of CP, given the reduced compliance of pericardium and its reduced stretching, diastolic pressures of the ventricles rapidly increase, and consequently, ventricular filling abruptly ceases during early to mid-diastole, when cardiac volume reaches the limit set by non-compliant pericardium. Thus, atrial emptying will be incomplete, leading to the increase of atrial and pulmonary/systemic venous pressure [4]. Systemic venous congestion results in hepatic congestion, peripheral edema, and ascites and, if long-standing, in cardiac cirrhosis and symptoms secondary to low cardiac output (**Figure 1**). As a matter of fact, although left ventricle (LV) ejection fraction is usually normal, the absolute reduction of diastolic filling, due to pericardial

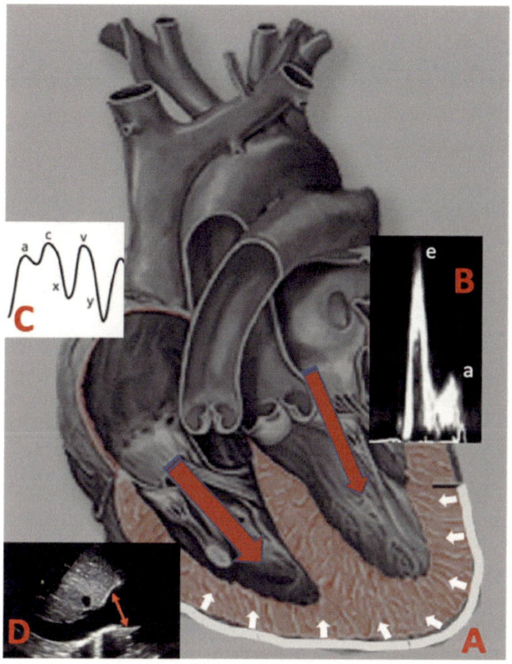

Figure 1.
Constrictive pericarditis physiology. During early to mid-diastole, ventricular filling (red arrows) is limited by pericardial thickness and incompliance (A) that resist to myocardial relaxation (white arrows) and, therefore, limiting ventricular preload to the early diastolic phase as showed by trans-mitral Doppler inflow pattern characterized by elevated and short "e"wave and a minor "a"wave (B) and sharp "y" descending wave at jugular vein pulse (C). Limitation to ventricular filling is, finally, associated to peripheral vein congestion as highlighted by dilation of inferior vena cava (D).

reduced compliance, leads to reduced cardiac output and, consequently, to fatigue and reduced functional class. Finally, physiologic reduction of intrathoracic pressure during inspiration acts on lungs and pulmonary veins, as usual, but will not be transmitted to the heart (*heart-lungs decoupling*) because of the limited heart diastolic compliance (myocardial relaxation, after reaching maximal diastolic volume limited by pericardium incompliance, fails to increase linearly with respect to negative intrathoracic pressure that usually drives a suction phenomenon). Consequently, whereas in normal hearts, trans-mitral flow increases during inspiration, as a consequence of this suction phenomenon, in patients with CP, it is reduced because pulmonary veins have a negative pressure with respect to the left atrium, resulting in a reduction of forward blood flow, and, finally, to LV diastolic filling [5]. This phenomenon clearly does not apply to right ventricle (RV) because inspiratory negative pressure is not applied to systemic veins (originating outside of thorax), and consequently, venous pressure is not lower than right atrial pressure so that diastolic filling of RV is less reduced than LV during inspiration (**Figure 2**). This right-left mismatch and ventricle inter-dependence secondary to thickened non-compliant pericardium (expansion of one ventricle occurs at expenses of the other one because both are into a rigid pericardial envelope) explain the reason why, as explained before, during inspiration, LV filling decreases whereas RV filling increases with secondary leftward interventricular septal shift (*septal bounce*). Conversely, during expiration, pulmonary vein pressure increases, driving forward blood flow and, therefore, increasing trans-mitral flow.

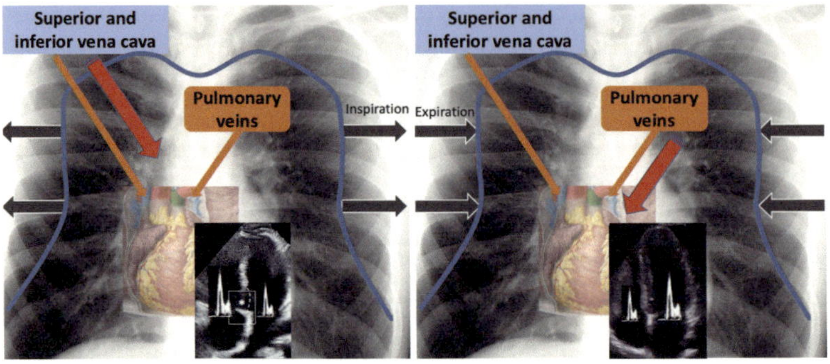

Figure 2.
Respiratory variations of ventricular filling pressures in constrictive pericarditis. During inspiration (left), thorax expansion is accompanied by a negative pressure transferred to lungs, pulmonary veins but not to the heart (because of uncompliant pericardium) and peripheral veins (outside of thorax). Pressure gradient from pulmonary veins to left atrium is reduced whereas gradient from vena cava to right atrium is increased (red arrow). Consequently, mitral inflow is reduced with respect to tricuspid flow and septum is shifted leftward (*). During expiration (right), a positive pressure is transferred on pulmonary veins driving the increase of gradient from pulmonary veins to left atrium (red arrow) and the increase of mitral inflow with respect to tricuspid inflow. As a consequence, septum returns to neutral position.

In this case, right ventricle filling, expressed as trans-tricuspid flow, decreases, and leftward interventricular septal deviation disappears [6].

4. Clinical "red flags"

When approaching a patient with CP, jugular venous pressure (JVP) increases, with specifically an abnormal increase during inspiration explicated by the incompliance of pericardium that impedes the venous blood, that usually increases because of suction inspiratory forces, to enter into the RV. This phenomenon (*Kussmaul's sign*) is opposite to normal condition when, during inspiration, usually JVP falls because more blood enters into RV. Moreover, JVP increase is associated to peculiar invasive pressure patterns (sharp descending *"y"* wave associated to rapid ventricle diastolic inflow and, if sinus rhythm is present, sharp descending *"x"* wave associated with late systolic inflow produced by atrial contraction) [7]. Consequently, the presence of peripheral edema, hepatomegaly, and, eventually, ascites are the cornerstone of clinical assessment. Finally, although the presence of restricted RV diastolic filling, most of all during inspiration when the higher venous return is not followed by an increase of ventricular filling, tricuspid flow increases with respect to mitral flow, explaining the presence, frequently, of a peripheral pulse markedly diminished, or even abolished, during ordinary or quiet inspiration (*paradoxical pulse*) secondary to the decrease of LV filling and, consequently, the drop of systolic pressure (>10 mmHg) during inspiration.

Finally, an essential clinical feature of CP is a *pericardial knock*, a high-pitched sound that occurs in early diastole and is best heard at the left sternal border and/or the cardiac apex [8].

5. Non-invasive imaging "red flags"

The essential technique for non-invasive assessment of CP is echocardiography that, moreover, is widely available and cost-saving. Therefore, it should be considered a first-line exam in patients with suspicion of CP. This is because, beside echocardiography,

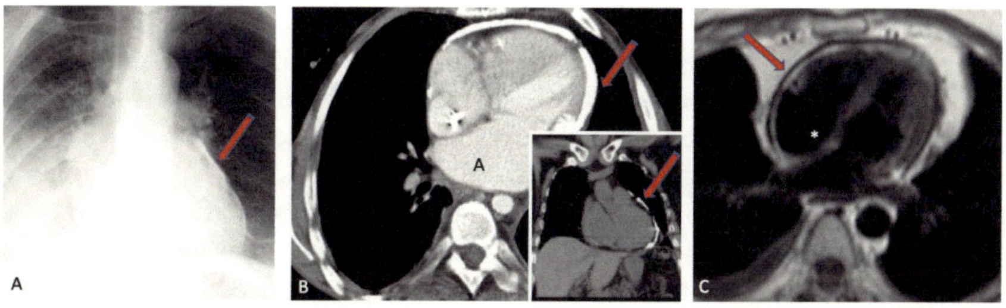

Figure 3.
Multimodality imaging of pericardial thickening and calcifications. Chest X Ray (A), Cardiac CT (B) and Cardiac MRI (C) revealing extensive pericardial calcifications (red arrows) suggesting pericardial constriction physiology. This is confirmed at Cardiac MRI by the presence of septal bounce phenomenon (*).

diagnosis of CP can be challenging with other techniques given the fact that there are no specific findings pathognomonic of pericardial constriction. As a matter of fact, atrial fibrillation at EKG can be a frequent finding in this subset of patients but, given its high prevalence in general population, lacks adequate specificity. On chest X-rays, pericardial calcification is not always seen and, when encountered, is not necessarily an expression of constrictive physiology [9]. Moreover, another useful but not specific marker of CP is pulmonary vascular congestion and redistribution on chest X-rays, secondary to the increase of LV filling pressures. Similarly, a CT scan permits to detect even small spots of pericardial calcification and minor increases of pericardial thickness (>2 mm) [10]. This applies also to MRI, without the need for iodinated contrast or ionizing radiations but with reduced accuracy than CT in detecting small calcifications and measuring thickness (**Figure 3**). Nonetheless, although pericardial morphology can be described precisely, physiologic repercussions of CP on ventricular diastole cannot be estimated directly and can be only presumed by hepatic venous congestion, ascites, and pleural effusions. A step-forward is obtained by Cine acquisition in which ventricular-wall-motion abnormalities and ventricular-contour distortion secondary to localized adhesions to pericardium (corresponding to areas of major pericardial calcifications) can be visualized, and moreover, ventricular inter-dependence can be derived by leftward interventricular septal shift during early diastole (*septal bounce*) [11].

Consequently, given the limitations of the aforementioned non-invasive techniques, echocardiography, when feasible (optimal ultra-sonographic window is not always available), is the exam of choice in this subset of patients. Importantly, a respirometer is mandatory in order to detect respirophasic changes of ventricular diastolic filling and septal movements [12].

Similar to Cine CT or MRI, first step of assessment of CP by echocardiography is the observation of thickened pericardium [13], with or without areas of tethering on myocardium, usually at the level of the right free wall, appreciated on sub-costal and apical 4-chambers views. In addition, septal bounce phenomenon during inspiration, a constant finding of CP, can be highlighted as a septal notch in an M-mode long-axis parasternal view [14].

Moreover, dilation of supra-hepatic and inferior vena cava is observed in a sub-costal view in almost all patients with CP.

Central role in echocardiographic assessment of CP is played by Doppler hemodynamic evaluation. Most of the times, Doppler findings can confirm constrictive physiology without the need for invasive confirmation. Mitral and tricuspid inflows are characterized by high early diastolic velocities (E wave) with short deceleration time and significant respiratory variations in 2/3rd of patients [15]. Mitral E wave variation

>25% (minimum at the end of inspiration) and tricuspid E wave variation>40% (maximum at the end on inspiration) are considered pathognomonic of CP, although absence of respiratory variation does not exclude the diagnosis (**Figure 3**). As a matter of fact, the presence of respiratory variations of mitral- and tricuspid-inflow-Doppler patterns alone can be present also without CP, like in patients with severe COPD due to higher respiratory variations of intra-thoracic pressures. Nonetheless, patients with COPD present a marked increase of inferior vena cava and supra-hepatic vein systolic forward flow velocity, whereas in patients with CP, this increase is blunted [16]. It is important to remember that in patients with CP, during inspiration, tricuspid flow is relatively increased with respect to mitral flow, but absolute flow is limited by pericardial constriction and, therefore, cannot increase significantly. A higher positive predictive value (96%) is offered by supra-hepatic-vein-Doppler pattern characterized by a decrease of expiratory diastolic forward velocities with large expiratory diastolic reversals.

Another useful parameter to detect CP is obtained by mitral annular tissue Doppler assessment of early diastolic velocity (e'wave), with evidence of *"annulus reversus"*, consistent with similar or slower lateral-wall relaxation with respect to septal wall (e'septal/e'lateral ratio > 0.91) when in normal conditions the opposite occurs, that has 95% of positive predictive value of CP [17]. Interestingly, absolute values of medial e'waves could be normal (septal e'wave > 9 cm/seg) or even increased (*annulus paradoxus*) despite the evidence of increased LV diastolic pressures (ratio E/e' > 13) [18]. This phenomenon is explicated by the predominance of longitudinal cardiac relaxation of septum during LV diastolic filling because lateral wall is frequently entrapped and tethered by thick and calcified pericardium. This marker, also, has 95% of positive predictive value for CP diagnosis (**Figure 4**). Unfortunately, both *annulus reversus* and *annulus paradoxus* are affected by a significant proportion of false negative results (50% and 57% of negative predictive values, respectively). Consequently,

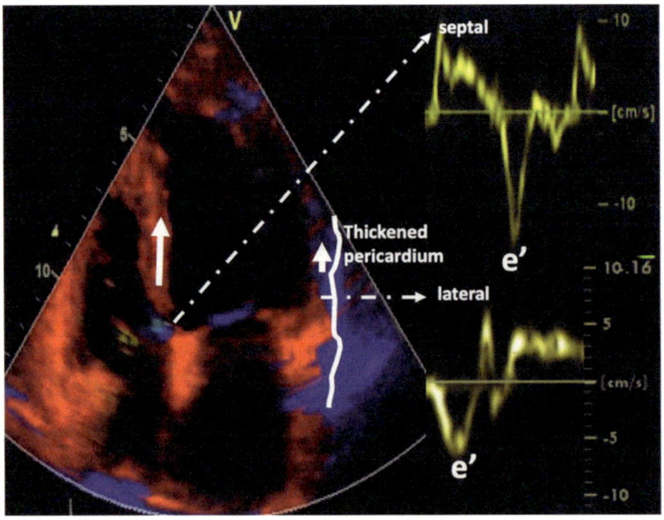

Figure 4.
Tissue Doppler characteristics of constrictive pericarditis. Contrary to normal physiology, in constrictive pericarditis lateral wall relaxation velocity (white arrow) during early diastole (e'wave) is usually is frequently reduced in comparison with septal e'wave (annulus reversus). This occurs because lateral wall is frequently entrapped and tethered by thick and calcified pericardium (white line). Moreover, although diastolic filling restriction is present, septal e'wave can be normal (> 8 cm/second) and can be used as a reliable marker of constriction in order to differentiate the latter with myocardial restriction (annulus paradoxus).

a multi-parametric approach is warranted to assess a patient with suspected CP, and in doubtful cases or when quality of echocardiography is sub-optimal (challenging acoustic window, respirometer not available), a multi-modal assessment with CT and/or MRI can be helpful in identifying calcifications, ventricular wall distortions, *septal bounce* during inspiration, and systemic vein congestion [19]. Finally, if doubts still persist, right- and left-heart catheterization is essential for invasive pressure measurement and, therefore, demonstration of equalization of RV and LV-end-diastolic pressures secondary to the non-compliance of pericardium, a common constraint for both ventricles.

6. Invasive hemodynamic assessment

Simultaneous right- and left-heart catheterization is currently the gold standard for the diagnosis of CP. Evidence of equalization of end-diastolic pressures (≤ 5 mmHg difference between right- and left-ventricle-end-diastolic pressures secondary to fixed pericardial volume and consequent ventricular interdependence) and the visualization

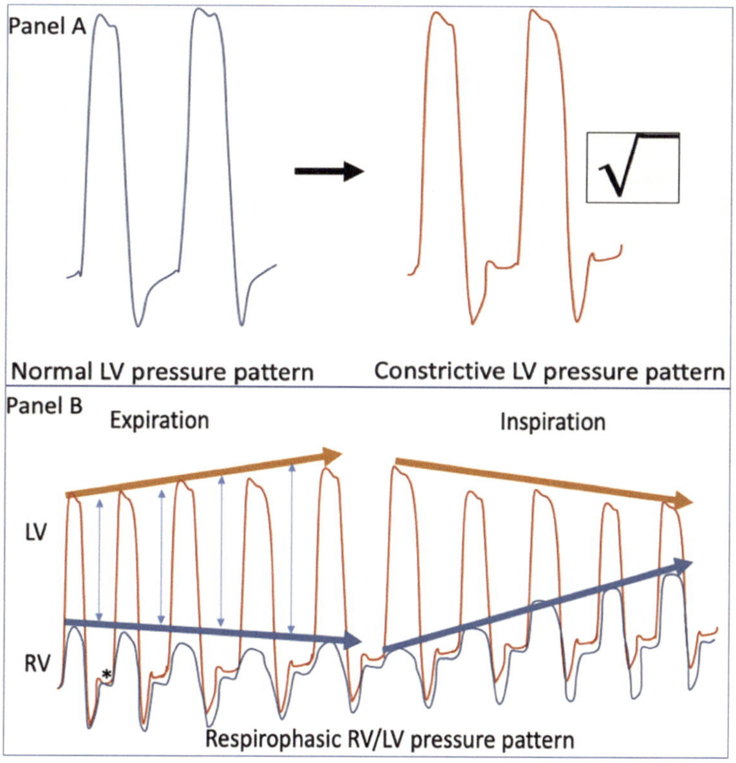

Figure 5.
Invasive pressure measurement characteristics of constrictive pericarditis. Constrictive physiology is characterized by sharp ventricular pressure increase after early diastolic inflow that, in comparison with normal hearts, is highlighted by a peculiar diastolic pressure curve morphology known as "square root" or "dip and plateau" (panel A). Moreover, ventricular interdependence (panel B) is another crucial marker of constriction and is demonstrated by equalization of end-diastolic pressures (≤ 5 mmHg difference between RV and LV end-diastolic pressures) secondary to fixed pericardial volume in which both ventricles are moving (*). The same mechanism, added to the dissociation between intra-cardiac and intrathoracic pressures, explains the evidence of RV and LV opposite respiratory variations (panel B). This is also a useful marker to distinguish pericardial constriction from myocardial restriction (in this case, LV pressure variates in the same manner whereas RV pressure remains stable as its preload is not influenced by intrathoracic pressure and both ventricles are independent from each other).

of "square root" or "dip and plateau" sign (secondary to sharp ventricular-pressure increase when pericardial constraining volume is reached immediately after early diastolic inflow) are considered the most important features for the diagnosis [20]. Another important marker of constriction is the presence of significant respiratory variations of LV and RV systolic and diastolic pressures as a consequence of dissociation between intracardiac and intrathoracic pressures (**Figure 5**). This has been quantified using the *systolic area index* (ratio of RV to LV systolic pressures × time area during inspiration). If >1.1 (RV pressure increasing while LV pressure decreasing during inspiration), it is highly suggestive of CP. Moreover, *Kussmaul's sign*, quantified as <5 mm Hg decrease in right atrial pressure during inspiration, is often encountered. It is worth mentioning that hypovolemia secondary to previous aggressive diuretic therapy can mask hemodynamic features described above. An important tip in these cases is to perform a fluid challenge with rapid infusion of saline (500–1000 ml over 5–10 min) before assessment [21]. Finally, not specific but important findings at invasive assessment are also the reduction of stroke volume (as per Frank-Starling effect secondary to reduced diastolic filling) and the maintenance of pulmonary artery pressures within or mildly above upper normal limit, explaining the higher prevalence of right instead of left heart-failure symptoms.

7. Constrictive versus restrictive physiology: differences and similarities

Clinical spectra of CP and RCM frequently overlap given the defect of diastolic ventricle filling that is common to both diseases. Anyway, as a specific treatment for each of them is present, a correct differential diagnosis is mandatory. RCM is characterized by increased myocardial stiffness and, therefore, increased ventricular filling pressures in both the systemic and pulmonary circulations with the increase of both mitral and tricuspid inflows during inspiration. Differently, CP is characterized by discordant respiratory flow variations in RV and LV (*ventricular interdependence*) (**Figure 5**), frequently accompanied by the *paradoxical pulse* sign and *septal bounce* pattern and, predominantly, by systemic venous congestion. That makes the presence of symptoms and signs of pulmonary edema and congestion more frequent in RCM than in CP. This phenomenon is also reflected by the presence of severe post-capillary pulmonary hypertension in RCM, whereas it is almost absent in patients with CP. Similarly, although both present a "square root" morphology of ventricular diastolic pressure, tele-diastolic pressures of LV and RV are usually equal in CP, whereas LV has usually a higher pressure (4–5 mmHg more) than RV in RCM [22]. Finally, from a clinical perspective, the presence of pericardial knock suggests CP diagnosis.

Moreover, non-invasive imaging modalities, like echocardiography, CT scan, and cardiac MRI, are helpful in the diagnostic process as the presence of pericardial calcifications and/or increased pericardial thickness suggest CP, whereas ventricular hypertrophy (with or without delayed gadolinium enhancement at MRI) and marked atrial enlargement suggest RCM. Finally, myocardial tethering by adhered pericardium is present in CP (absent in RCM) and is accompanied by LV shape deformations and/or reduced circumferential restoration and speckle-tracking examination with normal longitudinal restoration. On the contrary, in RCM, circumferential restoration is normal, whereas longitudinal restoration is reduced. Similarly, e'lateral is equal or slower than e'medial in CP (*annulus reversus*), whereas it is the opposite in patients with RCM (**Figure 4**). Medial e'wave is usually normal in patients with CP (reflecting the absence of myocardial disease), whereas it is reduced in patients with RCM (*annulus paradoxus*) [23]. Finally, in doubtful cases, endomyocardial biopsy could confirm or exclude RCM [24].

8. Treatment

Surgical pericardiectomy is the treatment of choice of CP with acceptable outcomes in the long-term [25–28]. Nonetheless, diuretic therapy is the first-line treatment of CP, often started even before proper diagnosis is obtained, and permits initially to control mild symptoms and reduce venous congestion. Unfortunately, as CP progresses, patients become refractory to diuretics and maintain an adequate cardiac output with compensatory sinus tachycardia. This is the reason why beta-adrenergic blockers, verapamil, and diltiazem should be avoided. In case of high-rate supraventricular arrhythmias, digoxin is the negative chronotropic agent of choice. In the specific subset of patients developing CP early (<3 months) after cardiac surgery, treatment with nonsteroidal anti-inflammatory agents, colchicine, and steroids for at least 3 months has been proposed. Predictors of success of this strategy are increased biomarkers of systemic inflammation (hsCRP) and evidence of significant pericardial inflammation visualized as intense delayed enhancement on MRI [29, 30]. Nonetheless, surgical pericardiectomy should not be delayed in case of failure of initial anti-inflammatory strategy as earlier surgery is associated with improved outcomes. In patients without ongoing acute pericardial inflammation or with long-standing symptoms, surgical pericardiectomy is the first-line treatment. Different surgical approaches have been described (on- versus off-pump, median sternotomy versus mini-invasive thoracotomy) without a clear benefit of one of them. Complete pericardiectomy, defined as extensive excision of pericardium up to superficial epicardium, if involved, anteriorly between the 2 phrenic nerves and from the great arteries superiorly to the diaphragm inferiorly, posteriorly between the left phrenic nerve to the left pulmonary veins,

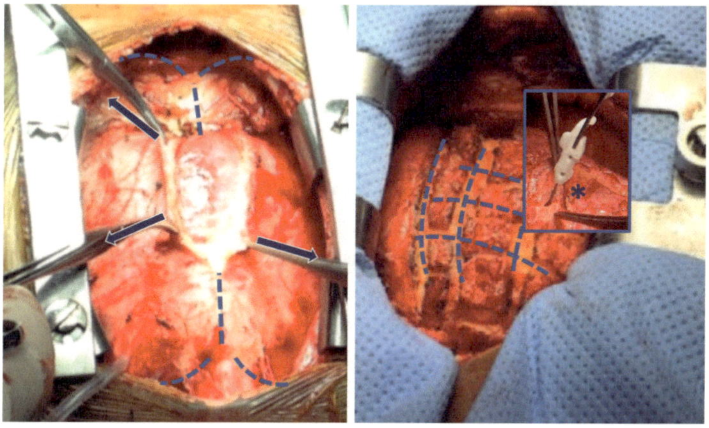

Figure 6.
Surgical approach to constrictive pericarditis. Complete pericardiectomy with extensive excision of pericardium anteriorly between the 2 phrenic nerves and from the great arteries superiorly to the diaphragm inferiorly (left panel) and posteriorly between the left phrenic nerve to the left pulmonary veins is considered the gold standard for treatment of CP. When extensive calcification is encountered, a less invasive approach with multiple transverse and longitudinal incisions up to the epicardial layer ("waffle" procedure) with the help of a dedicated ultrasonic scalpel (*) is considered a valid alternative (right panel).

including the diaphragmatic wall of left ventricle, is highly recommended. In case of severe calcification, it can be associated with ultrasound or laser debridement. Moreover, a less invasive approach with multiple transverse and longitudinal incisions on the epicardial layer (*"waffle"procedure*) has been proposed in patients with extensive calcific involvement of visceral pericardium and epicardium (**Figure 6**) [31, 32]. Despite long-standing experience in this procedure, pericardiectomy has a relatively high perioperative mortality rate (2–20%) associated with frequently reported low cardiac output. Predictors of poor perioperative outcomes are post-radiation CP, comorbidities (COPD, renal insufficiency, coronary artery disease, etc.), prior cardiac surgery, significant cardiac involvement (reduced LV systolic function, myocardial fibrosis/atrophy, severe tricuspid regurgitation), cardiopulmonary bypass, and poor functional status (New York Heart Association (NYHA) stage IV symptoms) [26]. Therefore, safety concerns about post-operative complications explain current indication to manage conservatively elderly healthy subjects, most of all in the presence of mild constriction, with pericardiectomy as a second-line therapy in case of progression. Similarly, patients at higher operative risk like elderly patients with severe symptoms and comorbidities are considered at prohibitively high risk, whereas radiation-induced CP is considered a relative contraindication to surgery.

9. Prognosis

Pericardiectomy, if performed early after diagnosis, is usually associated with acceptable quality of life. Symptomatic relief (associated with diastolic function recovery in up to 50% of cases) usually occurs immediately after surgery or, only in a small proportion of patients, after few months [27]. Long-term survival rates, unfortunately, remain moderately acceptable, despite surgical advances in the last decades, as reported in a meta-analysis of patients submitted to pericardiectomy [2] in which pooled all-cause 1-year and 5-year mortality rates after pericardiectomy were 17.4% and 32.7%, respectively. Interestingly, patients enrolled after 2000 had higher 1-year and 5-year all-cause mortality rates compared with before 2000 (19.8% vs. 10%, $p = 0.01$, and 49.4% versus 20%, $p < 0.001$, respectively). This possibly reflects the shift that occurred in the last decades toward more complex and recurrent etiologies of CP like cardiac surgery or mediastinal radiotherapy. As a matter of fact, patients with CP secondary to cardiac surgery have significantly higher risk of all-cause mortality after pericardiectomy when compared with patients with idiopathic etiology (HR: 2.15; 95% CI: 1.21 to 3.61, $p = 0.01$), with even worse outcomes when CP secondary to radiotherapy is compared with idiopathic etiology (HR: 3.21; 95% CI: 1.56 to 6.50, $p < 0.01$) [2]. Finally, pericardiectomy performed in patients with CP secondary to tuberculosis, the most common etiology observed in developing countries, has been recently reported to have similar outcomes with respect to other etiologies, although with more technical complexity in terms of increased operative time, more blood loss, and prolonged ICU and hospital stay [3].

10. Conclusion

Diagnosis of CP in the context of patients with signs and symptoms of heart failure can be challenging, and frequently, distinguishing it from RCM can be difficult. Firstly, thinking about CP when evaluating patients with diastolic dysfunction, most of all after cardiac surgery or mediastinal radiotherapy, is crucial to recall in our minds all the characteristics of CP and make it possible to address the correct diagnosis. CP should also be suspected when ventricular filling restrictions are observed few months after a tuberculosis infection, taking into account that tuberculosis is the first cause of CP in countries of sub-Saharan Africa and few countries of Asia.

Secondly, the use of multimodality imaging is the cornerstone for the diagnosis of CP and the evaluation of the extension of the disease and, finally, to guiding surgical treatment. In doubtful cases, we should not hesitate to ask for invasive pressure assessment, safe and diagnostic in the majority of the cases. Finally, long-terms results of surgery in patients with chronic end-stage disease are poor, most of all when CP is secondary to previous cardiac surgery or radiation therapy, also with less invasive surgical strategies like*"waffle"procedure.* Consequently, new therapeutic strategies are strongly warranted. Meanwhile, an early diagnosis could make the difference in the natural history of the disease and, therefore, should be actively promoted.

Acronyms and abbreviations

CP	constrictive pericarditis
RCM	restrictive cardio-myopathy
LV	left ventricle
RV	right ventricle
JVP	jugular venous pressure
CT	computed tomography
MRI	magnetic resonance imaging
hsCRP	high sensitive C reactive protein
NYHA	New York Heart Association

Author details

Francesco Maria Lauri
Mostoles University Hospital, Madrid, Spain

*Address all correspondence to: laurifm86@gmail.com

IntechOpen

© 2023 The Author(s). Licensee IntechOpen. This chapter is distributed under the terms of the Creative Commons Attribution License (http://creativecommons.org/licenses/by/3.0), which permits unrestricted use, distribution, and reproduction in any medium, provided the original work is properly cited.

References

[1] Adler Y, Charron P, Imazio M, et al. 2015 ESC Guidelines for the diagnosis and management of pericardial diseases: The task force for the diagnosis and management of pericardial diseases of the European Society of Cardiology (ESC). European Heart Journal. 2015;**36**:2921

[2] Tzani A, Doulamis IP, Tzoumas A, et al. Meta-analysis of population characteristics and outcomes of patients undergoing Pericardiectomy for constrictive pericarditis. The American Journal of Cardiology. 2021;**146**:120-127

[3] Benjamin SR, Mohammad A, Shankar R, et al. Does tuberculosis affect surgical outcomes following pericardiectomy for chronic constrictive pericarditis? Twelve years' experience from a tertiary care center in India. Indian Journal of Thoracic Cardiovascular Surgery. 2022;**38**(3):241-250

[4] Vistarini N, Chen C, Mazine A, et al. Pericardiectomy for constrictive pericarditis: 20 years of experience at the Montreal Heart Institute. The Annals of Thoracic Surgery. 2015;**100**:107

[5] Ling LH, Oh JK, Schaff HV, et al. Constrictive pericarditis in the modern era: Evolving clinical spectrum and impact on outcome after pericardiectomy. Circulation. 1999;**100**:1380-1386

[6] Nishimura RA, Tajik AJ. Evaluation of diastolic filling of left ventricle in health and disease: Doppler echocardiography is the clinician's Rosetta Stone. Journal of the American College of Cardiology. 1997;**30**:8-18

[7] Park JY, Eleid MF, Michelena HI. Abnormal neck veins. JAMA Cardiology. 2016;**1**:487-488

[8] Hancock EW. Differential diagnosis of restrictive cardiomyopathy and constrictive pericarditis. Heart. 2001;**86**:343-349

[9] Austin JH. The lateral chest radiograph in the assessment of nonpulmonary health and disease. Radiologic Clinics of North America. 1984;**22**:687-698

[10] Bull RK, Edwards PD, Dixon AK. CT dimensions of the normal pericardium. The British Journal of Radiology. 1998;**71**:923-925

[11] Gahide G, Granier M, Frapier JM. Effusive constrictive pericarditis: Functional and anatomical magnetic resonance findings. European Heart Journal. 2009;**30**:1371

[12] Welch TD, Ling LH, Espinosa RE, et al. Echocardiographic diagnosis of constrictive pericarditis: Mayo Clinic criteria. Circulation. Cardiovascular Imaging. 2014;**7**:526-534

[13] Ling LH, Oh JK, Tei C, et al. Pericardial thickness measured with transesophageal echocardiography: Feasibility and potential clinical usefulness. Journal of the American College of Cardiology. 1997;**29**:1317-1323

[14] Coylewright M, Welch TD, Nishimura RA. Mechanism of septal bounce in constrictive pericarditis: A simultaneous cardiac catheterisation and echocardiographic study. Heart. 2013;**99**:1376

[15] Hurrell DG, Nishimura RA, Higano ST, et al. Value of dynamic respiratory changes in left and right ventricular pressures for the diagnosis of constrictive pericarditis. Circulation. 1996;**93**:2007-2013

[16] Boonyaratavej S, Oh JK, Tajik AJ, et al. Comparison of mitral inflow and superior vena cava Doppler velocities in chronic obstructive pulmonary disease and constrictive pericarditis. Journal of the American College of Cardiology. 1998;**32**:2043-2048

[17] Reuss CS, Wilansky SM, Lester SJ, et al. Using mitral 'annulus reversus' to diagnose constrictive pericarditis. European Journal of Echocardiography. 2009;**10**:372-375

[18] Ha JW, Oh JK, Ling LH, et al. Annulus paradoxus: Transmitral flow velocity to mitral annular velocity ratio is inversely proportional to pulmonary capillary wedge pressure in patients with constrictive pericarditis. Circulation. 2001;**104**:976-978

[19] Verhaert D, Gabriel RS, Johnston D, et al. The role of multimodality imaging in the management of pericardial disease. Circulation. Cardiovascular Imaging. 2010;**3**:333

[20] Talreja DR, Nishimura RA, Oh JK, et al. Constrictive pericarditis in the modern era: Novel criteria for diagnosis in the cardiac catheterization laboratory. Journal of the American College of Cardiology. 2008;**51**:315-319

[21] Nishimura RA, Carabello BA. Hemodynamics in the cardiac catheterization laboratory of the 21st century. Circulation. 2012;**125**:2138-2150

[22] Sorajja P. Invasive hemodynamics of constrictive pericarditis, restrictive cardiomyopathy, and cardiac tamponade. Cardiology Clinics. 2011;**29**:191-199

[23] Rajagopalan N, Garcia MJ, Rodriguez L, et al. Comparison of new Doppler echocardiographic methods to differentiate constrictive pericardial heart disease and restrictive cardiomyopathy. The American Journal of Cardiology. 2001;**87**:86-94

[24] Leone O, Veinot JP, Angelini A, et al. 2011 consensus statement on endomyocardial biopsy from the Association for European Cardiovascular Pathology and the Society for Cardiovascular Pathology. Cardiovascular Pathology. 2012;**21**:245-274

[25] Gopaldas RR, Dao TK, Caron NR, Markley JG. Predictors of in-hospital complications after pericardiectomy: A nationwide outcomes study. The Journal of Thoracic and Cardiovascular Surgery. 2013;**145**:1227

[26] Tokuda Y, Miyata H, Motomura N, et al. Outcome of pericardiectomy for constrictive pericarditis in Japan: A nationwide outcome study. The Annals of Thoracic Surgery. 2013;**96**:571

[27] Biçer M, Özdemir B, Kan İ, et al. Long-term outcomes of pericardiectomy for constrictive pericarditis. Journal of Cardiothoracic Surgery. 2015;**10**:177

[28] Busch C, Penov K, Amorim PA, et al. Risk factors for mortality after pericardiectomy for chronic constrictive pericarditis in a large single-Centre cohort. European Journal of Cardio-Thoracic Surgery. 2015;**48**:e110

[29] Feng D, Glockner J, Kim K, et al. Cardiac magnetic resonance imaging pericardial late gadolinium enhancement and elevated inflammatory markers can predict the reversibility of constrictive pericarditis after antiinflammatory medical therapy: A pilot study. Circulation. 2011;**124**:1830-1837

[30] Mayosi BM, Ntsekhe M, Bosch J, et al. IMPI trial investigators. Prednisolone and Mycobacterium indicus pranii in tuberculous pericarditis.

The New England Journal of Medicine. 2014;**371**:1121-1130

[31] Azam S, Hoit BD. Treatment of pericardial disease. Cardiovascular Therapy. 2011;**29**:308

[32] Matsuura K, Mogi K, Takahara Y. Off-pump waffle procedure using an ultrasonic scalpel for constrictive pericarditis. European Journal of Cardio-Thoracic Surgery. 2015;**47**:e220

Section 3

Update on Diagnosis and Management of Recurrent Pericarditis

Chapter 4

Percutaneous Approach to Pericardial Disease Management

Jack Hartnett, Richard Armstrong, Lisa Brandon, Hani Jneid, Igor F. Palacios and Andrew O. Maree

Abstract

Percutaneous access of the pericardial space is increasingly sought. This is not only due to growing prevalence of pericardial effusions and cardiac tamponade, but also the emerging diagnostic and therapeutic potential of the pericardial space for mapping and ablation of arrhythmogenic circuits, biopsy, and drug delivery. Although increasingly performed, percutaneous pericardiocentesis remains a technically challenging procedure with potentially life-threatening complications. Consequently, management of patients with pericardial disease is highly complex. In this chapter we outline a step-by-step approach to percutaneous pericardiocentesis and the required specialised management of pericardial disease patients. Procedural complications are discussed along with their alleviating therapeutic strategies. Furthermore, we describe approaches to the prevention and management of recurrent pericardial effusion including diagnostic and therapeutic procedures such as percutaneous balloon pericardiotomy and intra-pericardial delivery of chemotherapeutics and sclerosing agents.

Keywords: pericardial effusion, cardiac tamponade, pericardiocentesis, percutaneous balloon pericardiotomy, pericardial disease management

1. Introduction

The pericardial space is a potential space contained between the inner visceral pericardium and the outer fibrous pericardium. In normal physiological states it contains up to 50 mL of serous fluid, which acts as a lubricant for the enclosed heart [1]. Similar to the pleural space, the pressure within the pericardial space varies with respiration driven changes in intra-thoracic pressure – ranging from – 5 cm of water during inspiration to +5 cm water during expiration. However, in certain pathological states, both the volume and pressure within the pericardial space can increase giving rise to haemodynamic compromise.

An increase in intra-pericardial volume and pressure is initially compensated for by the compliance of the pericardium [2]. However, when intra-pericardial pressure rises to equilibrate with or surpass intra-cardiac pressures (at approximately 15–20 mm Hg), right heart haemodynamic function is compromised. The underlying pathophysiology centres on excessive intra-pericardial pressures that cause compression of right heart chambers. Consequently, right ventricular filling is restricted and results in a reduction in cardiac output, increased systemic venous pressures and ultimately cardiac tamponade.

Cardiac tamponade is a clinical diagnosis characterised by the concurrent presence of three non-specific clinical signs known as Beck's Triad. This comprises hypotension, distended neck veins and 'distant muffled' heart sounds on auscultation [3]. Although cardiac tamponade is classically taught as a potentially fatal medical emergency requiring immediate intervention, in practice, the presentation is a spectrum ranging from more subtle asymptomatic persistent hypotension (often refractory to intravenous fluid resuscitation) to life-threatening circulatory collapse.

Clinical severity is not only determined by the volume of fluid within the pericardial space, but also the rate at which it accumulates. Rapidly developing pericardial effusions are more likely to cause cardiac tamponade at smaller fluid volumes than slowly accumulating effusions [2]. In rapidly accumulating pericardial effusions, the pericardium remains relatively stiff resulting in a rapid rise in intra-pericardial pressure. In comparison, slow progressive effusions allow for adaptive stretching of the pericardium over time and thus result in lower intra-pericardial pressures for longer.

Echocardiography is crucial to the assessment of any patient with suspected pericardial effusion and/or cardiac tamponade [4]. It can be performed quickly at the bedside to confirm cardiac tamponade in an emergency setting. Although less convenient, haemodynamic assessment during invasive catheterisation can also provide important diagnostic information. **Boxes 1** and **2** outline key echocardiographic and haemodynamic findings in cardiac tamponade.

Definitive management is drainage of the excess pericardial fluid. This is most commonly performed via percutaneous pericardiocentesis which involves insertion of a needle through the skin into the pericardial sac to drain the effusion and relieve haemodynamic compromise on the heart. In this chapter we outline a step-by-step guide to percutaneous pericardiocentesis along with the peri-procedural management of pericardial patients. Novel techniques to prevent and alleviate recurrent pericardial effusions – such as percutaneous balloon pericardiotomy and intra-pericardial chemotherapeutics – are also discussed.

- Presence of a pericardial effusion
- Right atrial collapse in late diastole
- Right ventricular free wall collapse in early diastole
- Increase in E-wave velocity across tricuspid valve during inspiration
- Decrease in E-wave velocity across mitral valve during inspiration
- Inspiratory decrease and expiratory increase in diastolic pulmonary venous forward flow
- Dilated inferior vena cava without inspiratory collapse

Box 1.
Key echocardiographic findings in cardiac tamponade.

- Elevated right atrial pressure
- Elevated intra-pericardial pressure (very similar to right atrial pressure)
- Elevation and equalisation of left–right ventricular filling pressure
- Loss of y descent of the right atrial pressure waveform
- Arterial pulsus paradoxus (i.e., an inspiratory decrease in excess of 10 mmHg in systolic blood pressure)

Box 2.
Key haemodynamic findings in cardiac tamponade.

2. Percutaneous pericardiocentesis

2.1 Indications

The clinical utility of percutaneous pericardiocentesis cannot be understated. It is both diagnostic – providing pericardial fluid for analysis of cell counts, cytology, culture etc. – as well as therapeutic – reducing intra-pericardial pressures and improving right ventricular filling and cardiac output. However, as subsequently outlined, it is a technically challenging procedure with potential life-threatening complications. As such, there are a narrow range of indications for percutaneous pericardiocentesis (**Box 3**) [5].

Timing of percutaneous pericardiocentesis depends on the degree of haemodynamic deterioration and the rapidity with which compromise has developed. Echocardiographic features, aetiology of the underlying effusion and risk–benefit ratio of the procedure (e.g. presence of concurrent coagulopathy) must be considered.

Among patients with life-threatening circulatory collapse, immediate intervention is required. However, the clinical scenario is more complex when haemodynamic compromise is progressive. Percutaneous pericardiocentesis may be deferred to facilitate appropriate planning but these patients remain at high risk of clinical deterioration. Numerous scoring systems have been developed to aid clinicians in determining the timing of intervention. *Halpern et al.,* developed a pericardial effusion scoring

- Cardiac tamponade
- Suspected bacterial pericarditis (including tuberculous pericarditis)
- Suspected neoplastic pericarditis
- Moderate to large pericardial effusions not responsive to medical therapy
- Chronic (persisting longer than 3 months) large pericardial effusion (> 20 mm on echocardiography in diastole)

Box 3.
Indications for percutaneous pericardiocentesis.

index to predict need for pericardiocentesis among patients with haemodynamically stable moderate-to-large pericardial effusions [6]. More recently, the ESC Working Group on Myocardial and Pericardial Diseases published a novel triage system based on aetiology, clinical presentation and diagnostic imaging findings [7]. A combined score of six or greater requires urgent pericardiocentesis. In cases of a score less than six, intervention can be delayed for up to 12–24 hours to facilitate planning. Of note, these recommendations are not based on a body of published data but rather on expert opinion. As such randomised studies are required to validate this triage system.

In the absence of clinical haemodynamic compromise, echocardiographic evidence of cardiac tamponade is not a clear indication for intervention as recent evidence suggests echocardiographic findings of 'pre-tamponade physiology' may be over-sensitive [4]. Consequently, despite near ubiquity of echocardiographic assessment, the decision to proceed with pericardiocentesis is primarily a clinical one.

2.2 Contraindications

Percutaneous pericardiocentesis is potentially life-saving and as such there are no absolute contraindications. It is, however, a technically challenging procedure with potential complications. The decision to intervene mandates risk–benefit analysis. Furthermore, surgery may offer a superior alternative to percutaneous intervention in some clinical scenarios (**Box 4**).

Haemopericardium secondary to aortic dissection, trauma (iatrogenic or otherwise) or ventricular free wall rupture post myocardial infarction are clear indications for emergency cardiothoracic surgery [8]. Furthermore surgical repair should not be

- Haemopericardium secondary to type A aortic dissection
- Traumatic haemopericardium
- Haemopericardium secondary to post-myocardial infarct ventricular free wall rupture
- Bleeding diathesis
    - Use of anticoagulants
    - Raised INR/APTT/PT
    - Platelet count <50,000
- Recurrent pericardial effusions
- Purulent pericardial effusions
- Small pericardial effusions that warrant drainage
- Loculated pericardial effusions
- Posteriorly located pericardial effusions difficult to access percutaneously

Box 4.
Situations warranting special consideration before performing pericardiocentesis.

delayed by attempted percutaneous pericardiocentesis. Only in cases where surgery is delayed or the patient is too unstable for transfer to theatre should percutaneous intervention for controlled drainage of small amounts of haemopericardium be considered [9]. Surgery is also preferred for unstable septic patients with purulent pericardial effusions and in cases of loculated effusions [5].

Surgery offers numerous advantages that include access to large pericardial tissue samples for histopathological analysis, the ability to insert large bore drains (particularly important in purulent pericardial effusions) and the ability to drain complex loculated effusions. However, outside of the scenarios outlined above, surgical risk may outweigh benefit. In particular, general anaesthesia may cause hypotension and circulatory collapse in patients with restrictive cardiac physiology [10].

Percutaneous pericardiocentesis for diagnostic purposes alone is generally not recommended. Aetiology of an effusion can usually be determined based on clinical presentation, laboratory results and imaging without requiring pericardial fluid samples for analysis. Evidence suggests that in approximately 60% of pericardial effusions there is an identifiable underlying cause [11]. In the case of small effusions that do not meet criteria for therapeutic drainage, procedural risk is high.

Similarly percutaneous drainage is not recommended for idiopathic pericardial effusions without haemodynamic compromise. Published data indicate that such effusions respond well to anti inflammatory therapy or resolve spontaneously [5].

3. Performing a percutaneous pericardiocentesis

3.1 Preparation

Informed consent must be obtained from the patient with capacity. The procedure itself must be explained along with the indication and potential complications (**Box 5**) [12–14].

- Monitor ECG signal from aspiration needle
    - ST segment elevation/premature ventricular contractions (PVCs) suggest epicardial irritation or puncture
    - PR segment elevation/premature atrial contractions (PACs) suggest entry into right atrium
- Monitor pressure
    - Intrapericardial pressure tracing observed (right ventricular pressure waveform suggests entry into right ventricle)
- Inject agitated saline and observe for bubbles arriving in pericardial space with echocardiography
- Inject contrast under fluoroscopic screening
- Advance an 0.035-inch J wire and observe it wrapping around heart using fluoroscopy

Box 5.
Techniques for confirming needle/catheter placement in the pericardial space.

The procedure should be performed in the catheterisation laboratory either under echocardiographic [15] or fluoroscopic guidance [16]. In emergency settings percutaneous pericardiocentesis in a controlled planned environment may not be possible and the procedure may have to be performed at the bedside under echocardiographic guidance alone.

Monitoring of heart rate, blood pressure and oxygen saturations along with continuous electrocardiographic (ECG) monitoring is required. Echocardiography facilitates needle tip visualisation and confirms entry into the pericardial space. A resuscitation trolley should be available at the bedside to pre-empt life-threatening complications. Furthermore, a sonographer and nurse should be present during the procedure to provide assistance.

3.2 Patient positioning

The patient should be positioned head-up at a 30–45° angle to allow pooling of the fluid to the inferior surface of the pericardial sac. The objective of patient positioning is to minimise the distance between the skin surface and the target fluid contained within the pericardial space.

3.3 Selecting an entry site

Prior to creation of a sterile field with a drape, the most appropriate entry site should be determined using echocardiography. The entry site should be the shortest distance from the skin to the pericardial fluid – thus minimising the risk of damage to intervening structures. Once the optimal entry site has been selected, the proceduralist should note the distance in centimetres from the probe to the pericardial fluid. This acts as an approximate guide for the distance in which the needle tip should be inserted to achieve access to the pericardial fluid.

The classical entry site is sub-xiphoid as usually the fluid accumulates along the inferior surface of the pericardial sac under gravity. However, the rise in the use of echocardiographic visualisation has enabled alternative access sites (e.g. apical, parasternal) to be used safely depending on the clinical scenario. Distance to the pericardial space is greater with the sub-xiphoid approach compared to other entry sites and risk of damage to adjacent structures (e.g. liver, peritoneal cavity) is higher, likelihood of iatrogenic pneumothorax is lower compared to an apical or parasternal approach. Recent evidence supports echocardiography-guided entry site selection with numerous observational studies reporting fewer peri-procedural complications compared to a traditional sub-xiphoid approach [12, 13, 15, 17].

3.4 Aseptic technique

A strict aseptic technique must be adhered to such that introduction of iatrogenic infection into the pericardial space is avoided. The skin around the proposed entry site is first cleaned with aseptic solution prior to the application of a drape to create the sterile field. Additional sterile drapes placed over the lower abdomen and lower limbs reduce risk of inadvertent contamination.

3.5 Local anaesthetic

One percent lignocaine is infiltrated into the skin at entry site. Local anaesthetic should also be injected into the deeper subcutaneous tissues along the proposed route to minimise intra-procedural pain. Care must be taken when applying lignocaine to ensure it is not infiltrated into small intervening blood vessels.

3.6 Access to the pericardial space

A needle is inserted at a 90° angle to the skin along the planned trajectory. As outlined above, the most common entry point is sub-xiphoid. However, with the advent of more advanced imaging techniques, alternative entry points are increasingly common – particularly in instances of loculated pericardial effusions [18]. The needle is advanced at an angle of 15–30° toward the left shoulder such that it passes beneath the inferior costal margin.

Continuous aspiration should be attempted during insertion to avoid inadvertent entry into vasculature and to confirm entry into the pericardial space. Further local anaesthetic can be infiltrated into the subcutaneous tissues intermittently during entry as additional intra-procedural analgesia.

3.7 Approaches for confirming entry into pericardial space

3.7.1 'Blind'

In emergency situations at high risk of immediate patient demise, percutaneous pericardiocentesis may need to be performed 'blind'. In such cases, ECG monitoring and continuous needle aspiration during insertion should be utilised to confirm pericardial space entry. The commencement of fluid drainage from the inserted needle is suggestive of entry. However, a sanguineous aspirate may pose a dilemma for the clinician as it may be unclear whether this is due to a haemorrhagic pericardial effusion or myocardial puncture. The development of ST segment elevation on continuous ECG monitoring is suggestive of needle over-advancement leading to myocardial injury [19].

3.8 Echocardiography

Since the development of echocardiography-guided pericardiocentesis in 1979, the technique has rapidly become standard of care [17]. The approach can either be performed under continuous echocardiographic surveillance, in which the needle tip is visualised throughout its trajectory from skin to pericardial space [20], or via the echocardiography assisted technique, in which the probe is used only to confirm entry into the space post insertion [17].

Regardless of approach subtype, correct position can be determined by injecting 5–10 mL of agitated saline through the needle and visualising bubbles arriving into the pericardial space. The presence of bubbles within the cardiac chambers is suggestive of needle over-advancement into the myocardium and should alert the clinician to withdraw. Inability to visualise bubbles can either be due to extra-cardiac position of the needle tip or presence of a very large pericardial effusion which hampers visualisation. To distinguish between the two potential aetiologies more agitated saline should be injected and the pericardial space visualised from an alternative echocardiographic window.

3.9 Fluoroscopy

Fluoroscopy guided pericardiocentesis is performed in the catheterisation laboratory - most commonly for iatrogenic pericardial effusions that occur during interventional procedures or cardiac surgery [21, 22]. Injection of contrast through the needle tip followed by radiographic imaging can be used to assess needle tip position relative to the pericardial space. Should the position be correct, contrast will pool in the dependent portion of the pericardial space. Alternatively, a 0.035-inch J-wire can be inserted through the needle. It should be seen to curl around the heart silhouette on radiographic imaging if the needle tip is in the pericardial space. Guidewire position should be confirmed in two orthogonal planes (e.g., lateral and antero-posterior). Passage outside of this silhouette indicates an extra-pericardial location.

Fluoroscopy guidance is limited by radiation exposure to both patient and clinician along with the requirement to be performed in the catheterisation laboratory.

3.10 Computed tomography (CT)

In recent years computed tomography (CT) guided pericardiocentesis has emerged as a viable alternative technique for select indications such as cardiac effusions which are often posteriorly located and difficult to visualise with echocardiography [23]. The procedure involves a planning CT scan to delineate pericardial anatomy, subsequent needle insertion through the marked trajectory followed by a single CT scan post procedure to confirm needle entry. This technique is not performed under continuous CT imaging.

There are clear drawbacks to CT guided pericardiocentesis – lack of continuous imaging during insertion, radiation exposure and prolonged procedure time (median time is 65 minutes per procedure in one study [24]). However, despite these shortcomings, CT guidance does have clinical utility. It is particularly useful for cases of difficult-to-access loculated pericardial effusions or for access to 'dry' pericardial spaces (i.e., do not contain an effusion) for interventional procedures.

3.10.1 Drainage catheter placement

The drainage catheter is inserted via Seldinger-technique. A 0.035-inch J wire is inserted through the needle into the pericardial space. If resistance to insertion is encountered, the J-wire should not be forced. Instead troubleshooting should begin to identify the source of resistance. Once the J-wire is correctly and securely positioned, the insertion needle can be removed. A 6–8 Fr dilator is then inserted over the wire to dilate the entry tract for subsequent placement of the 6–8 Fr pigtail drainage catheter. Appropriate positioning of the drainage catheter can be proven via the various techniques outlined above.

The end of the 6–8 Fr pigtail drainage catheter is connected to a three-way tap so that pericardial fluid can be initially drained into a 50 mL Leur-lock syringe and subsequently transferred into the drainage bag. The drain is usually sutured to the skin to prevent dislodgement – particularly in cases of likely prolonged drainage time.

4. Post pericardiocentesis management

Management of patients post percutaneous pericardiocentesis should occur in a specialised cardiac care unit (CCU) at a tertiary level medical centre where possible (**Box 6**). It is a technically challenging life-saving procedure with potential complications.

A chest X-ray (CXR) should be obtained immediately post procedure to exclude an iatrogenic pneumothorax. Regular vital sign recording along with clinical observation should be undertaken to ensure early detection of complications such as haemodynamic collapse, pericardial decompression syndrome or iatrogenic introduction of infection.

Appropriate care of the drainage catheter is essential. The catheter can either be left on continuous free drainage or intermittent aspiration. Intermittent aspiration every 4–6 hours via the three-way valve system is often preferred in clinical practice due to the lower risk of luminal occlusion [25]. The drainage system should be flushed with sterile heparinised saline between aspirations to preserve patency.

The volume of pericardial fluid drained should be recorded at regular intervals. Drainage of greater than 450 mL in the immediate post insertion setting should be avoided due to the higher risk of pericardial decompression syndrome [26].

The drain should be removed when less than 25 mL of fluid is drained in a 24-hour period [25]. Prior to removal an echocardiogram should be performed to ensure

- Close vital sign monitoring and clinical observation for development of complications
- Post-procedure chest x-ray (CXR) to exclude pneumothorax
- Analgesia (usually with non-steroidal anti-inflammatory agents) as required for pericardial pain
- Catheter drainage can be either free drainage or intermittent aspiration
- Record volume draining at regular intervals
- Strict aseptic technique for catheter manipulation
- Flush drainage catheter with heparinised saline every 6–8 hours
- Minimise duration of catheter stay to reduce risk of infection
- Remove catheter as soon as appropriate or when volume draining is less than 25 mL in 24 hour period
- Remove drainage catheter in event of fever or septic clinical deterioration
- Perform echocardiogram to determine residual pericardial effusion size prior to removing drainage catheter
- Surveillance echocardiogram at appropriate intervals following catheter removal
- Immediate echocardiogram in event of haemodynamic deterioration

Box 6.
Post-pericardiocentesis management.*

adequate interval echocardiographic improvement. In the event of haemodynamic instability post pericardial drain removal an immediate echocardiogram should be performed to assess for evidence of cardiac tamponade [25].

5. Complications of percutaneous pericardiocentesis

Although considered a high-risk procedure, complication rates for echocardiography guided or fluoroscopy guided percutaneous pericardiocentesis are low. Multiple large scale retrospective observational studies report total complication rates of up to 4.7–6.2% [12, 27]. Importantly, procedural success rates are high. In one study involving 1127 echocardiography guided pericardiocentesis procedures over 21 years, procedural success rate was 97% and did not change over the study period [12]. However, it must be noted, these analyses were performed from patient cohorts across a timespan of decades in large tertiary level institutions with considerable expertise. As such real-life complication rates may be higher when performed for emergency indications in lower volume centres by less experienced clinicians.

In comparison, 'blind' percutaneous pericardiocentesis is associated with a life-threatening complication rate of 20% and a mortality risk of up to 6% [19]. Consequently, imaging guided pericardiocentesis is the gold standard and a 'blind' procedure should only be performed in life-threatening emergency settings when no alternative is readily available.

Complications of percutaneous pericardiocentesis include death due to iatrogenic damage to the myocardium or adjacent structures. Myocardial or coronary artery puncture can result in haemopericardium and worsening tamponade. Haemopericardium can initially be clinically silent or present as either a tamponade refractory to drainage or worsening bloody pericardial drain output. Iatrogenic peri-procedural haemopericardium occurs in less than 1% of cases and is an indication for emergent cardiothoracic surgery [19].

Accidental puncture of surrounding structures can also have deleterious consequences. Vascular damage (including puncture of the intercostal vessels or internal mammary vessels) can lead to significant blood loss. Piercing of the lung parenchyma can result in a pneumothorax while accidental intra-peritoneal puncture (most likely with a sub-xiphoid approach) can lead to intra-abdominal organ damage. The most commonly involved intra-abdominal structure is the liver, however, cases of hollow viscus perforation and inferior vena cava perforation have been reported [28, 29].

Incidence of bacterial infection introduction into the pericardial space is low. As such there is no consensus on use of prophylactic antibiotics in the peri-procedural setting.

Arrhythmias in the peri-procedural setting is also a concern. All patients should be on continuous electrocardiographic monitoring during the procedure and during post-procedural observation in the cardiac care unit [30]. ST segment elevation during pericardiocentesis is an indicator of possible myocardial needle puncture while persistent ST segment elevation post procedure is suggestive of potential coronary artery injury leading to myocardial injury [19, 31]. Vasovagal bradycardia is common post pericardiocentesis. Although generally self-limiting, there have been documented fatalities secondary to vasovagal hypotension [32].

Pericardial decompression syndrome, although it has multiple aliases, it is broadly defined as an acute deterioration in haemodynamics that results in hypotension and pulmonary oedema post an uncomplicated pericardiocentesis procedure [33–35]. It is estimated to occur in 5% of cases [36]. Although there is some limited data to suggest it occurs more frequently in malignant effusions, there is no strong predisposition for any particular effusion aetiology [36]. The underlying pathophysiology has not been fully elucidated, however, there are multiple proposed mechanisms. One theory suggests increased right ventricular venous return post decompression results in septal bowing and a consequent drop-off in left ventricular stroke volume leading to pulmonary oedema [34, 37, 38]. Another proposed mechanism involves left ventricular myocardial stunning secondary to pericardial compression induced coronary ischaemia [36, 39]. Judicious drainage of the pericardial effusion to allow haemodynamic re-equilibration is recommended to avoid the development of pericardial decompression syndrome. The European Society of Cardiology recommends rapid drainage of the fluid volume required to clinically alleviate tamponade but that subsequent fluid drainage should be no more than 1 L in 24 hours to allow haemodynamic re-equilibration [5].

6. Recurrent pericardial effusions

The natural course of a pericardial effusion can be unpredictable. To prevent fluid re-accumulation and to promote adherence of the pericardial layers, the drain should not be removed until output is <30 mL in a 24-hour period. In cases at high risk of effusion recurrence, prolonged drainage is a Class IB recommendation from the European Society of Cardiology as it has been shown to reduce recurrence rates [5]. Despite this, recurrent pericardial effusion post-pericardiocentesis is common. It is particularly frequent among malignant pericardial effusions which have a recurrence rate as high as 31–62% [40, 41].

There are multiple therapeutic options for the management of recurrent pericardial effusions including repeated percutaneous pericardiocentesis, intra-pericardial administration of sclerosing agents or chemotherapeutics or creation of a pericardial 'window' - either through open cardiothoracic surgery, a video assisted thorascopic approach (VATS) approach or percutaneous balloon pericardiotomy.

There is no guideline or consensus on the approach for interventional management of recurrent effusions as there is a paucity of evidence directly comparing management strategies.

6.1 Surgical pericardial window

Although not the scope of this chapter, surgical intervention for recurrent pericardial effusion is common – either via drainage through a pericardial window or surgical pericardiectomy. Access to the pericardium can be obtained either via an open thoracotomy, an open sub-xiphoid incision or VATS approach [42].

Multiple small retrospective single institution analyses have reported that while initial success and diagnostic yield is similar between surgical and percutaneous pericardiocentesis, the complication rate and re-accumulation rates are lower with surgical intervention [43, 44]. It must be noted that these studies included first presentation and recurrent pericardial effusions and both malignant and non-malignant aetiologies. In some studies, there may be a selection bias toward surgical intervention as the cohort also included post-operative pericardial effusions following cardiothoracic surgery. A recent published analysis of 44,637 non-surgically related pericardial effusion cases managed either surgically or percutaneously has reported higher mortality and re-intervention rates with percutaneous intervention but increased risk of post-procedural complications and longer hospital admissions with surgery [45].

6.2 Percutaneous balloon pericardiotomy

Percutaneous balloon pericardiotomy is a less-invasive alternative for the management of recurrent pericardial effusion. It is usually reserved for patients with recurrent malignant effusions who are unfit for surgical intervention or in whom the in-hospital post-operative period would significantly impact their remaining limited quality of life.

First described by *Palacios et al.*, in 1991, percutaneous balloon pericardiotomy is similar to a conventional percutaneous pericardiocentesis procedure [46]. It is performed in a cardiac catheterisation laboratory under either fluoroscopic or echocardiographic guidance. A sub-xiphoid approach is used and the area pre-infiltrated with local anaesthetic prior to incision. A stiff 0.038-inch wire with a pre-shaped broad curved tip is advanced into the pericardial space via a needle or through a pre-existing pericardial drain catheter. Position is confirmed via either echocardiography or fluoroscopy. A 10French dilator is advanced over the wire to pre-dilate the skin and subcutaneous tissues and then removed. A balloon-dilating catheter is then advanced over the wire under fluoroscopic guidance until it straddles the parietal pericardium. A 30 × 20 mm diameter balloon is used, but use of the Inoue balloon (Torray International America Inc., Houston, TX, USA) has also been described. It is essential the proximal end of the balloon is beyond the skin to prevent pericardio-cutaneous fistula formation. The position of the balloon is confirmed via insufflation with a contrast – saline mix. Insufflation is repeated until the waist formed by the parietal pericardium on the balloon visually disappears. The balloon-dilating catheter is then replaced with a pericardial drain catheter.

Post-procedural management is similar to percutaneous pericardiocentesis described above. However, intra-operative and post-operative pain is greater with balloon pericardiotomy – primarily due to purposeful stretching of the nociceptive fibre rich parietal pericardium [47]. Consequently, pre-medication with analgesics and regular pain scores is essential to the care of a balloon pericardiotomy patient.

The previously listed complications of percutaneous pericardiocentesis can also be seen with percutaneous balloon pericardiotomy. However, post-procedural left sided pleural effusion is more common following balloon pericardiotomy. This is believed to be due to balloon insufflation induced creation of a pericardiopleural window which allows the recurrent effusion to drain into the more resorptive pleural space. In one retrospective analysis by *Ziskind et al.* involving 50 cases of balloon pericardiotomy, a post-procedural pleural effusion was seen in all cases and eight required thoracocentesis mediated drainage [47]. Post-operative pneumothorax also appears to occur more commonly with balloon pericardiotomy.

Although usually reserved for oncology patients with poor operative fitness, percutaneous balloon pericardiotomy is an effective alternative to surgical intervention with procedural success rates of 85–100% documented in retrospective studies [48, 49]. However, patient prognosis is poor. Median survival post procedure in these patients is reported up to 3.3 months [47]. The poor survival was primarily driven by underlying malignancy since peri-procedural mortality rates were low (approximately 0–1%) [48].

Overall, there remains a paucity of evidence surrounding percutaneous balloon pericardiotomy. The 2015 ESC guidelines for the diagnosis and management of pericardial diseases do not recommend balloon pericardiotomy for neoplastic effusions but rather "in rare cases of recurrent effusion" [5].

6.3 Intra-pericardial delivery of therapeutics

Intra-pericardial administration of therapeutics is a potential percutaneous intervention which can be performed once percutaneous access has been obtained and the effusion has been drained.

The most common indication is for delivery of sclerosing agents, which drive inflammation and fibrosis of the visceral and parietal layers – thus eliminating the potential space for fluid to re-accumulate. A variety of chemotherapeutic or sclerosing agents have been employed in the past. These include tetracyclines [50], bleomycin [51], cisplatin [52, 53] and thiotepa [54, 55].

Intra-pericardial instillation of sclerosing agents such as talc has no proven recurrence reduction benefit over other approaches including balloon pericardiotomy and surgical intervention. Although it has lower peri-procedural risks, specific complications include severe retrosternal chest pain (likely due to the induction of constrictive pericarditis), atrial arrhythmias or electrocardiographic changes on monitoring suggestive of sub-pericardial or epicardial injury [56, 57].

The 2015 ESC guidelines on the diagnosis and management of pericardial disease recommend intra-pericardial instillation of chemotherapeutics as part of the management of large neoplastic pericardial effusions [5]. It has been shown to reduce recurrence for lung and breast malignancy associated pericardial effusions [52–54]. Chemotherapy choice should be tailored to the specific malignancy – cisplatin is more effective for lung malignancy [52, 53] and thiotepa more beneficial in breast cancer [54].

7. Pericardial complications of Catheter Ablation

Catheter ablation of atrial fibrillation is an established therapy however pericardial effusion is a common complication that occurs in up to 14% of cases [58]. The majority of effusions are mild and asymptomatic and resolve spontaneously within a month. However pericardial tamponade may occur in up to 1% of cases and is usually related to traumatic transseptal puncture [59].

Ischaemic and non-ischaemic cardiomyopathy and infiltrative myocardial disease may be complicated by ventricular tachycardia. Treatment with catheter ablation is increasingly employed with improved outcome. While an endocardial approach is most common, presence of epicardial re-entrant circuits can result in treatment failure and necessitate an epicardial approach. This approach can be percutaneous or surgical and improves procedural success but major complication rates in certain sub-groups, such as post infarct patients, may be as high as 14%. Complications include haemopericardium, right ventricular puncture and may necessitate emergent cardiac surgery [60].

8. Conclusions

Incidence of cardiac tamponade is rising due to the increasing prevalence of pericardial access for electrophysiological intervention and cardiothoracic surgery.

Fortunately, percutaneous pericardiocentesis is a safe and effective intervention for the management of this potentially life-threatening clinical syndrome. However, the field of percutaneous pericardial intervention has significantly expanded beyond pericardiocentesis alone. More complex interventional techniques including balloon pericardiotomy and intra-pericardial instillation of chemotherapeutic agents have emerged, particularly in the management of recurrent malignant pericardial effusions.

Conflict of interest and funding

None.

Author details

Jack Hartnett[1], Richard Armstrong[1], Lisa Brandon[1], Hani Jneid[2], Igor F. Palacios[3] and Andrew O. Maree[1*]

1 Department of Cardiology, St James's Hospital, Dublin, Ireland

2 Division of Cardiology, Department of Internal Medicine, University of Texas Medical Branch (UTMB), Galveston, United States

3 Division of Cardiology, Massachusetts General Hospital, Harvard Medical School, Boston, United States

*Address all correspondence to: amaree@tcd.ie

IntechOpen

© 2023 The Author(s). Licensee IntechOpen. This chapter is distributed under the terms of the Creative Commons Attribution License (http://creativecommons.org/licenses/by/3.0), which permits unrestricted use, distribution, and reproduction in any medium, provided the original work is properly cited.

References

[1] Hoit BD. Anatomy and physiology of the pericardium. Cardiology Clinics. 2017;**35**(4):481-490. DOI: 10.1016/j.ccl.2017.07.002

[2] Shabetai R. Pericardial effusion: Haemodynamic spectrum. Heart. 2004; **90**(3):255-256. DOI: 10.1136/hrt.2003.024810

[3] Beck CS. Two cardiac compression triads. Journal of the American Medical Association. 1935;**104**(9):714-716. DOI: 10.1001/jama.1935.02760090018005

[4] Alerhand S, Carter JM. What echocardiographic findings suggest a pericardial effusion is causing tamponade? The American Journal of Emergency Medicine. 2019;**37**(2): 321-326. DOI: 10.1016/j.ajem.2018.11.004 Epub 2018 Nov 17

[5] Adler Y, Charron P, Imazio M, Badano L, Barón-Esquivias G, Bogaert J, et al. 2015 ESC guidelines for the diagnosis and management of pericardial diseases: The task force for the diagnosis and management of pericardial diseases of the European society of cardiology (ESC) endorsed by: The European association for cardio-thoracic surgery (EACTS). European Heart Journal. 7 Nov 2015;**36**(42):2921-2964. DOI: 10.1093/eurheartj/ehv318. Epub 2015 Aug 29. PMID: 26320112; PMCID: PMC7539677

[6] Halpern DG, Argulian E, Briasoulis A, Chaudhry F, Aziz EF, Herzog E. A novel pericardial effusion scoring index to guide decision for drainage. Critical Pathways in Cardiology. 2012;**11**(2): 85-88. DOI: 10.1097/HPC.0b013e318254a5ca

[7] Ristić AD, Imazio M, Adler Y, Anastasakis A, Badano LP, Brucato A, et al. Triage strategy for urgent management of cardiac tamponade: a position statement of the European society of cardiology working group on myocardial and pericardial diseases. European Heart Journal. 2014;**35**(34): 2279-2284

[8] Isselbacher EM, Cigarroa JE, Eagle KA. Cardiac tamponade complicating proximal aortic dissection. Is pericardiocentesis harmful? Circulation. 1994;**90**(5):2375-2378. DOI: 10.1161/01.cir.90.5.2375

[9] Cruz I, Stuart B, Caldeira D, et al. Controlled pericardiocentesis in patients with cardiac tamponade complicating aortic dissection: Experience of a centre without cardiothoracic surgery. European Heart Journal: Acute Cardiovascular Care. 2015;**4**(2):124-128. DOI: 10.1177/2048872614549737

[10] Madhivathanan PR, Corredor C, Smith A. Perioperative implications of pericardial effusions and cardiac tamponade. BJA Education. 2020; **20**(7):226-234. DOI: 10.1016/j.bjae.2020.03.006 Epub 2020 Jun 12

[11] Sagristà-Sauleda J, Mercé J, Permanyer-Miralda G, Soler-Soler J. Clinical clues to the causes of large pericardial effusions. The American Journal of Medicine. 2000;**109**(2): 95-101. DOI: 10.1016/s0002-9343(00)00459-9

[12] Tsang TS, Enriquez-Sarano M, Freeman WK, Barnes ME, Sinak LJ, Gersh BJ, et al. Consecutive 1127 therapeutic echocardiographically guided pericardiocenteses: Clinical profile, practice patterns, and outcomes spanning 21 years. Mayo Clinic Proceedings. 2002;**77**(5):429-436. DOI: 10.4065/77.5.429

[13] Cho BC, Kang SM, Kim DH, Ko YG, Choi D, Ha JW, et al. Clinical and echocardiographic characteristics of pericardial effusion in patients who underwent echocardiographically guided pericardiocentesis: Yonsei Cardiovascular Center experience, 1993-2003. Yonsei Medical Journal. 2004;**45**(3):462-468. DOI: 10.3349/ymj.2004.45.3.462

[14] Duvernoy O, Borowiec J, Helmius G, Erikson U. Complications of percutaneous pericardiocentesis under fluoroscopic guidance. Acta Radiologica. 1992;**33**(4):309-313

[15] Callahan JA, Seward JB, Tajik AJ. Cardiac tamponade: Pericardiocentesis directed by two-dimensional echocardiography. Mayo Clinic Proceedings. 1985;**60**(5):344-347. DOI: 10.1016/s0025-6196(12)60541-2

[16] Maisch B, Ristić AD, Seferović PM, Tsang TS. Interventional Pericardiology: Pericardiocentesis, Pericardioscopy, Pericardial Biopsy, Balloon Pericardiotomy and Intrapericardial Therapy. Heidelberg: Springer Medizin Verlag; 2011

[17] Tsang TS, Freeman WK, Sinak LJ, Seward JB. Echocardiographically guided pericardiocentesis: Evolution and state-of-the-art technique. Mayo Clinic Proceedings. 1998;**73**(7):647-652. DOI: 10.1016/S0025-6196(11)64888-X

[18] Cooper JP, Oliver RM, Currie P, Walker JM, Swanton RH. How do the clinical findings in patients with pericardial effusions influence the success of aspiration? British Heart Journal. 1995;**73**(4):351-354. DOI: 10.1136/hrt.73.4.351

[19] Kumar R, Sinha A, Lin MJ, Uchino R, Butryn T, O'Mara MS, et al. Complications of pericardiocentesis: A clinical synopsis. International Journal of Critical Illness and Injury Science. 2015; **5**(3):206-212. DOI: 10.4103/2229-5151.165007

[20] Maggiolini S, Gentile G, Farina A, De Carlini CC, Lenatti L, Meles E, et al. Safety, efficacy, and complications of pericardiocentesis by real-time echo-monitored procedure. The American Journal of Cardiology. 2016;**117**(8):1369-1374. DOI: 10.1016/j.amjcard.2016.01.043. Epub 2016 Feb 3

[21] Alp I, Ugur M, Selcuk I, Ulucan AE, Temizkan V, Yilmaz AT. Safety pericardiocentesis with fluoroscopy following cardiac surgery. Annals of Thoracic and Cardiovascular Surgery. 2019;**25**(3):158-163. DOI: 10.5761/atcs.oa.18-00188. Epub 2019 May 8

[22] Kim EY, Won JH, Kim J, Park JS. Percutaneous pericardial effusion drainage under ultrasonographic and fluoroscopic guidance for symptomatic pericardial effusion: A single-center experience in 93 consecutive patients. Journal of Vascular and Interventional Radiology. 2015;**26**(10):1533-1538. DOI: 10.1016/j.jvir.2015.07.014 Epub 2015 Aug 19

[23] Klein SV, Afridi H, Agarwal D, Coughlin BF, Schielke LH. CT directed diagnostic and therapeutic pericardiocentesis: 8-year experience at a single institution. Emergency Radiology. 2005;**11**:353-363

[24] Neves D, Silva G, Morais G, et al. Computed tomography-guided pericardiocentesis - A single-center experience. Revista Portuguesa de Cardiologia. 2016;**35**:285-290

[25] De Carlini CC, Maggiolini S. Pericardiocentesis in cardiac tamponade:

Indications and practical aspects. e-Journal of Cardiology Practice. 2017;**15**:3-5

[26] Pradhan R, Okabe T, Yoshida K, Angouras DC, DeCaro MV, Marhefka GD. Patient characteristics and predictors of mortality associated with pericardial decompression syndrome: A comprehensive analysis of published cases. European Heart Journal Acute Cardiovascular Care. 2015;**4**(2): 113-120. DOI: 10.1177/204887261 4547975 Epub 2014 Sep 1

[27] Pennacchioni A, Nanni G, Sgura FA, Imberti JF, Monopoli DE, Rossi R, et al. Percutaneous pericardiocentesis for pericardial effusion: Predictors of mortality and outcomes. Internal and Emergency Medicine. 2021;**16**(7): 1771-1777. DOI: 10.1007/s11739-021-02642-x Epub 2021 Feb 22

[28] Emmert MY, Frauenfelder T, Falk V, Wilhelm MJ. Emergency pericardiocentesis: A word of caution! Accidental transhepatic intracardiac placement of a pericardial catheter. European Journal of Cardio-Thoracic Surgery. 2012;**42**:e31-e32

[29] Dabbah S, Fischer D, Markiewicz W. Pericardiocentesis ending in the superior vena cava. Catheterization and Cardiovascular Interventions. 2005;**64**: 492-494

[30] Bishop LH Jr, Estes EH Jr, Mcintosh HD. The electrocardiogram as a safeguard in pericardiocentesis. Journal of the American Medical Association. 1956;**162**(4):264-265. DOI: 10.1001/jama.1956.02970210 004002

[31] Hsia HH, Kander NH, Shea MJ. Persistent ST-segment elevation following pericardiocentesis: Caution with thrombolytic therapy. Intensive Care Medicine. 1988;**14**(1):77-79. DOI: 10.1007/BF00254130

[32] Cotoi S, Moldovan D, Caraşcă E, Incze A, Herszenyi L, Podoleanu D. Sinus node dysfunction occurring immediately after pericardiocentesis. Physiologie. 1987;**24**(1):63-68

[33] Glasser F, Fein AM, Feinsilver SH, Cotton E, Niederman MS. Non-cardiogenic pulmonary edema after pericardial drainage for cardiac tamponade. Chest. 1988;**94**:869-870

[34] Vandyke WH Jr, Cure J, Chakko CS, Gheorghiade M. Pulmonary edema after pericardiocentesis for cardiac tamponade. The New England Journal of Medicine. 1983;**309**:595-596

[35] Sabzi F, Faraji R. Predictors of post pericardiotomy low cardiac output syndrome in patients with pericardial effusion. Journal of Cardiovascular and Thoracic Research. 2015;7:18-23

[36] Prabhakar Y, Goyal A, Khalid N, Sharma N, Nayyar R, Spodick DH, et al. Pericardial decompression syndrome: A comprehensive review. World Journal of Cardiology. 2019;**11**(12):282-291. DOI: 10.4330/wjc.v11.i12.282

[37] Braverman AC, Sundaresan S. Cardiac tamponade and severe ventricular dysfunction. Annals of Internal Medicine. 1994;**120**:442

[38] Wolfe MW, Edelman ER. Transient systolic dysfunction after relief of cardiac tamponade. Annals of Internal Medicine. 1993;**119**:42-44

[39] Skalidis EI, Kochiadakis GE, Chrysostomakis SI, Igoumenidis NE, Manios EG, Vardas PE. Effect of pericardial pressure on human coronary circulation. Chest. 2000;**117**: 910-912

[40] Kim SH, Kwak MH, Park S, Kim HJ, Lee HS, Kim MS, et al. Clinical characteristics of malignant pericardial effusion associated with recurrence and survival. Cancer Research and Treatment. 2010;**42**(4):210-216. DOI: 10.4143/crt.2010.42.4.210 Epub 2010 Dec 31

[41] Laham RJ, Cohen DJ, Kuntz RE, Baim DS, Lorell BH, Simons M. Pericardial effusion in patients with cancer: Outcome with contemporary management strategies. Heart. 1996;**75**:67-71

[42] Langdon SE, Seery K, Kulik A. Contemporary outcomes after pericardial window surgery: Impact of operative technique. Journal of Cardiothoracic Surgery. 2016;**11**:73

[43] Horr SE, Mentias A, Houghtaling PL, Toth AJ, Blackstone EH, Johnston DR, et al. Comparison of outcomes of pericardiocentesis versus surgical pericardial window in patients requiring drainage of pericardial effusions. The American Journal of Cardiology. 2017; **120**(5):883-890. DOI: 10.1016/j.amjcard.2017.06.003 Epub 2017 Jun 15

[44] Saltzman AJ, Paz YE, Rene AG, Green P, Hassanin A, Argenziano MG, et al. Comparison of surgical pericardial drainage with percutaneous catheter drainage for pericardial effusion. The Journal of Invasive Cardiology. 2012; **24**(11):590-593

[45] Pan CS, Mabeza RM, Tran Z, Lee C, Hadaya J, Sanaiha Y, et al. Pericardiocentesis or surgical drainage: A national comparison of clinical outcomes and resource use. PLoS One. 2022;**17**(4): e0267152. DOI: 10.1371/journal.pone.0267152

[46] Palacios I, Tuzcu E, Sizkind A. Percutaneous balloon pericardial window for patients with malignant pericardial effusion and tamponade. Catheterization and Cardiovascular Diagnosis. 1991;**22**:244-249

[47] Ziskind AA, Pearce AC, Lemmon CC, Burstein S, Gimple LW, Herrmann HC, et al. Percutaneous balloon pericardiotomy for the treatment of cardiac tamponade and large pericardial effusions: Description of technique and report of the first 50 cases. Journal of the American College of Cardiology. 1993;**21**(1):1-5. DOI: 10.1016/0735-1097(93)90710-i

[48] Sigusch HH, Geisler W, Surber R, Schönweiß M, Gerth J. Percutaneous balloon pericardiotomy: Efficacy in a series of malignant and nonmalignant cases. Scandinavian Cardiovascular Journal. 2022;**56**(1):331-336. DOI: 10.1080/14017431.2022.2111463

[49] Herron C, Forbes TJ, Kobayashi D. Single center experience of pediatric percutaneous balloon pericardiotomy. Cardiology in the Young. 2021;**31**(2): 212-215. DOI: 10.1017/S1047951120003686 Epub 2020 Nov 3

[50] Davis S, Sharma SM, Blumberg ED, Kim CS. Intrapericardial tetracycline for the management of cardiac tamponade secondary to malignant pericardial effusion. The New England Journal of Medicine. 1978;**299**(20): 1113-1114. DOI: 10.1056/NEJM197811162992006

[51] Lambert A, Salleron J, Kieffer A, Raymond P, Geoffrois L, Gavoille C. Intrapericardial instillation of bleomycin prevents recurrence of malignant pericardial effusions: Series of 46 cases and comprehensive literature review. Bulletin du Cancer. 2020;**107**(7–8): 756-762. DOI: 10.1016/j.bulcan.2020.04.010 Epub 2020 Jun 5

[52] Tomkowski WZ, Filipecki S. Intrapericardial cisplatin for the management of patients with large malignant pericardial effusion in the course of the lung cancer. Lung Cancer. 1997;**16**(2–3):215-222. DOI: 10.1016/s0169-5002(96)00631-9

[53] Maisch B, Ristić AD, Pankuweit S, Neubauer A, Moll R, Neoplastic pericardial effusion. Efficacy and safety of intrapericardial treatment with cisplatin. European Heart Journal. 2002; **23**(20):1625-1631. DOI: 10.1053/euhj.2002.3328

[54] Martinoni A, Cipolla CM, Cardinale D, Civelli M, Lamantia G, Colleoni M, et al. Long-term results of intrapericardial chemotherapeutic treatment of malignant pericardial effusions with thiotepa. Chest. 2004; **126**(5):1412-1416. DOI: 10.1378/chest.126.5.1412

[55] Colleoni M, Martinelli G, Beretta F, Marone C, Gallino A, Fontana M, et al. Intracavitary chemotherapy with thiotepa in malignant pericardial effusions: An active and well-tolerated regimen. Journal of Clinical Oncology. 1998;**16**(7):2371-2376. DOI: 10.1200/JCO.1998.16.7.2371

[56] Kunitoh H, Tamura T, Shibata T, et al. A randomised trial of intrapericardial bleomycin for malignant pericardial effusion with lung cancer (JCOG9811). British Journal of Cancer. 2009;**100**:464-469

[57] Shephard FA, Morgan C, Evans WK, Ginsberg JF, Watt D, Murphy K. Medical management of malignant pericardial effusion by tetracycline sclerosis. The American Journal of Cardiology. 1987; **60**(14):1161-1166

[58] Chierchia GB, Capulzini L, Droogmans S, Sorgente A, Sarkozy A, Müller-Burri A, et al. Pericardial effusion in atrial fibrillation ablation: A comparison between cryoballoon and radiofrequency pulmonary vein isolation. Europace. 2010;**12**(3):337-341. DOI: 10.1093/europace/eup422 Epub 2010 Jan 6

[59] Lellouche N, Sebag FA, Elbaz N, Hassine M, Chaachoui N, Teiger E, et al. Acute pericardial effusion following atrial fibrillation ablation: Characteristics and relationship with arrhythmia recurrences. Archives of Cardiovascular Diseases. 2011;**104**(8–9):450-457. DOI: 10.1016/j.acvd.2011.05.005 Epub 2011 Aug 27

[60] Sarkozy A, Tokuda M, Tedrow UB, Sieria J, Michaud GF, Couper GS, et al. Epicardial ablation of ventricular tachycardia in ischemic heart disease. Circulation. Arrhythmia and Electrophysiology. 2013;**6**(6):1115-1122. DOI: 10.1161/CIRCEP.113.000467 Epub 2013 Oct 9

Section 4

Clinicopathologic Phenotypes of Pericarditis Associated with Small-Vessel Vasculitis

Chapter 5

Current Treatment of ANCA Vasculitis

Yosra Bouattour, Mouna Snoussi and Zouhir Bahloul

Abstract

Anti-neutrophil cytoplasmic antibody (ANCA)-associated vasculitis (AAV) constitute a group of necrotizing systemic vasculitis with preferential involvement of small- to medium-sized vessels. None treated; they are considered as a life-threatening illness by their renal, cardiac and neurologic damages. Therefore, treatment is usually aggressive, with high-dose corticosteroid therapy combined with immunosuppressive drugs in the major part of cases. New biologic drugs have been introduced such as rituximab. In this chapter, we will present the update and recent advances in the treatment of AAV.

Keywords: ANCA vasculitis, granulomatosis with polyangiitis (Wegener's), microscopic polyangiitis, Eosinophilic granulomatous with polyangiitis, treatment

1. Introduction

Anti-neutrophil cytoplasmic antibody (ANCA)-associated vasculitis (AAV) constitute a group of necrotizing systemic vasculitis with preferential involvement of small- to medium-sized vessels. They represent serious disorders, and three clinical subtypes are involved: granulomatosis with polyangiitis (GPA; formerly Wegener's disease), microscopic polyangiitis (MPA) and eosinophilic GPA (EGPA; formerly Churg Strauss Syndrome). They share similar pathogenic mechanisms, and most patients have only one ANCA serotype detected in their serum [1, 2]. Non-treated, they were considered as fatal or life-threatening illnesses. In the last two decades, better knowledge of pathogenic mechanisms and progression in classification criteria improved therapeutic management [3–5]. Treatment is usually aggressive, with high-dose corticosteroid therapy combined with immunosuppressive drugs in the major part of cases. New biologic drugs have been introduced such as rituximab [4]. In this chapter, we will present the update and recent advances in the treatment of AAV.

2. Pathogenesis of ANCA-associated vasculitis:new paths for intervention

The etiology of AAV remains poorly understood, and research on their pathogenesis focuses on the role of ANCAs themselves [4].

2.1 Role of ANCA antibodies and neutrophils

ANCAs, which represent autoantibodies directed against neutrophil cytoplasmic proteins, recognize a range of antigens. Only two relevant protein targets are identified, called proteinase 3 (PR3) and myeloperoxidase (MPO). These proteins are found in the primary granules of neutrophils and are involved in defense against microbes [5].

During AAV and in small vessels, a pathological and sustained interaction occurs between ANCA and abnormally activated neutrophils. Thus, in the systemic form of GPA, ANCAs recognize PR3 in about 75% of cases. Whereas MPO-ANCA is more commonly associated with MPA (60%) and EGPA (50%) [5–7].

Experimental and clinical data provide evidence that ANCAs and neutrophils are the key players in pathogenesis. In response to inflammation or infection, neutrophils exposed to cytokines (interleukin 1, tumor necrosis factor α...) or complement C5a become primed with movement of MPO and PR3 from primary granules to the cell surface. ANCAs bind to these autoantigens on the neutrophil surface. Neutrophils become activated and bind to vascular endothelium, resulting in tissue damage.

2.2 Role of the complement system, cellular and humeral immunity

The pathogenesis of AAV also involves [5–8]

A. Activation of the alternative complement pathway responsible for the amplification of neutrophil-ANCA activation.

B. Monocytes and macrophages: in the formation of the classic GPA granuloma.

C. B and T lymphocytes: in the occurrence of endothelial damage and granuloma formation.

D. Eosinophilic polynuclear cells: The blood level of eosinophils can be high in the various vasculitis. These cells have cytotoxic granules that can contribute to cardiac involvement and vascular damage as seen in EGPA [7].

2.3 Predisposing factors for ANCA-associated vasculitis

A. Environmental factors:

- Pesticides, asbestos, smoke and silica.
- A number of therapeutic agents are responsible for drug-induced AAV such as propylthiouracil, benzylthio-uracil and hydralazine ... [5].
- Chronic carriage of staphylococcus aureus which is reported to be a risk factor for relapse in GPA.

B. Genetic predisposition: Familial cases of AAV have been reported and predisposing HLA haplotypes such as HLA DPB1 [8].

3. Classification and prognostic score of ANCA-associated vasculitis

3.1 Classification criteria of ANCA-associated vasculitis:

3.1.1 Granulomatosis with polyangiitis

Granulomatosis with polyangiitis (GPA), formerly named Wegner's disease, is characterized by vessel wall inflammation, peri- and extra-vascular granulomatosis. Its annual incidence is 10.2 cases per million people, and its prevalence is between 24 and 150 cases per million people [9]. Caucasians are the most affected persons according to researches conducted in Europe [10]. GPA is diagnosed at an age of 35–55 years with no gender predominance.

This disease involves mainly upper and lower airways, ear nose throat sphere and kidney. Nasosinus involvement occurs in 70–100% of patients as epistaxis, nasal septum deformation or perforation [11, 12]. Lungs manifestations affect 50–90% of the patients as lung nodules, cavitations, pleuritis and/or alveolar hemorrhages. Renal involvement affects 40–100% of patients as abnormalities in urine sediment and renal failure. Other systemic manifestations may include arthralgia, anorexia, weight loss, ocular involvement (episcleritis, uveitis, retinal thrombosis, orbital pseudotumor...) myocarditis [11]. Recently, a new criteria set has been approved and validated by the American College of Rheumatology (ACR) and the European Alliance of Associations for Rheumatology (EULAR). The aim of the classification criteria is to differentiate GPA from other types of small- or medium-vessel vasculitis (**Table 1**) [13].

A limited form of GPA is defined by the presence of upper airways and/or pulmonary involvement without alveolar hemorrhage. There is no renal involvement or life-threatening conditions.

A diffuse or severe form of GPA is known by the presence of a severe renal dysfunction and/or progressive alveolar hemorrhage and/or life-threatening organ involvement.

Clinical criteria	
Nasal involvement: bloody discharge ulcers, crusting, congestion, blockage, septal defect/ perforation	+3
Cartilaginous involvement (inflammation, of ear or nose cartilage, hoarse voice or stridor, endobronchial involvement or saddle nose deformity	+2
Conductive or sensorineural hearing loss	+1
Laboratory, imaging and biopsie criteria	
Positive test for cytoplasmic antineutrophil cytoplasmic antibodies (c ANCA) or antiproteinase 3 (anti-PR3) antibodies	+5
Pulmonary nodules, mass or cavitation on chest imaging	+2
Granuloma, extravascular granulomatous inflammation or giant cells on biopsy	+2
Pauci-immune glomerulonephritis on biopsy	+1
Positive test for perinuclear antineutrophil cytoplasmic antibodies (pANCA) or antimyeloperoxidase (anti-MPO) antibodies	−1
Blood eosinophil count ≥1* 10^9 /liter	−4

Table 1.
2022 American college of rheumatology (ACR)/European alliance of associations for rheumatology [13].

3.1.2 Eosinophilic granulomatosis with polyangiitis

Eosinophilic granulomatosis with polyangiitis (EGPA) formerly known as Churg–Strauss syndrome is a rare systemic small-vessel vasculitis associated with asthma and eosinophilia. EGPA is the least common systemic vasculitis among AAV with an annual incidence of 4.2 cases per million people and a prevalence of 10.7 per million people [14]. It affects people aged between 40 and 60 years with no gender predominance or ethnic predisposition [15, 16]. In 1990, ACR defined the classification criteria for EGPA including asthma, eosinophilia >10%, neuropathy, non-fixed lung infiltrates, paranasal sinus abnormalities and extravascular eosinophils on biopsy (**Table 2**) [17]. EGPA should be suspected in a patient with an adult-onset asthma and multiple systemic manifestations (asymmetric neuropathy, purpura or skin ulcers, cardiac, pulmonary and/or renal involvement ...). Laboratory data show mainly peripheral eosinophilia (>1500 cells/μL) correlated with the disease activity [18]. MPO-ANCA with perinuclear Immunofluorescence (pANCA) are noted in 50% [5]. Histologic findings confirm the leukocytoclastic vasculitis with eosinophilic granulomas in different biopsy sites (lung, kidney...).

3.1.3 Microscopic polyangiitis

MPA is a systemic necrotizing vasculitis with a pneumo-renal tropism. Capillaritis is the cause of its main feature including alveolar hemorrhage and rapidly progressive glomerulonephritis. The annual incidence of MPA is about 5.8 cases per million people [14]. MPA affects older patients compared to other AAV (between 50 and 60 years) [19]. Some studies suggest that increased life expectancy may contribute to the increased incidence of this disease [20]. Men are more frequently affected than women [14]. Other clinical manifestations may include general signs (fever, weight loss) in 70% of patients, skin lesions as vascular pupura, peripheral neuropathy, liver dysfunction and gastrointestinal manifestations. MPO-ANCA are detected in about 50% of cases, but its absence does not exclude its diagnosis [5]. Histological data allow the differentiation of MAP from other AAV. This entity is characterized by the absence of eosinophilic tissue infiltration found in GEPA and granulomas found mainly in GPA but also in GEPA.

3.1.4 Five-factor score: a prognosis score of ANCA-vasculitis

The five-factor score (FFS) for AAV is used to evaluate prognosis at diagnosis of the vasculitis. The following factors were significantly combined with higher five-year mortality: age > 65 years, cardiac involvement, renal insufficiency (creatinine ≥150 μmol/L) and gastrointestinal symptoms. The presence of each was scored +1

1. Asthma
2. Eosinophilia >10%
3. Neuropathy (mono- or poly-neuropathy)
4. Non-fixed pulmonary infiltrates
5. Paranasal sinus abnormalities
6. Extravascular eosinophil infiltration on biopsy
At least four of the six ACR criteria are required.

Table 2.
ACR classification of EGPA [17].

Age > 65 years
Cardiac insufficiency
Renal insufficiency (Creatinemia>150 μmol/L)
Gastrointestinal involvement
Absence of ear, nose and throat manifestation for GPA and EGPA.
One point for each of these five items when present.

Table 3.
Revised 2011 Five-Factor score in AAV [21].

point. Whereas ear, nose and throat (ENT) involvement, affecting patients with GPA and EGPA, were associated with a lower risk of death. Their absence was accorded +1 point (**Table 3**) [21].

4. Treatment of granulomatosis with polyangiitis

The choice of treatments in GPA depends on several forms of the disease (limited vs. diffuse), patient's age, his overall physiological state and in particular his renal function. At present, the choice of treatment according to the immunological profile (ANCA-PR3, ANCA-MPO or ANCA-negative) remains a subject of controversy [22].

4.1 Remission induction therapy

Regardless the clinical form of GPA, the treatment is based on a combination of corticosteroids with immunosuppressant drug or rituximab. Corticosteroids are used at a dose of 1 mg/kg/day, preceded by methylprednisolone pulses (7.5 to 15 mg/kg/day) in severe or active cases. The choice of the immunosuppressant drug depends on the clinical form and extent of the disease [22, 23].

4.2 Non-severe or limited forms of granulomatosis with polyangiitis

Methotrexate, rituximab and cyclophosphamide are effective at inducing remission the limited form of GPA. Although, methotrexate is currently recommended in this patient group [24]. The weekly dose is 0.3 mg/kg. According to the NORAM study, its efficacy is comparable to that of cyclophosphamide with a lower risk of infection. Also, mycophenolate mofetil (MMF) is effective as an induction therapy for the limited form of GPA with satisfactory results. Rituximab may be used for patients with recurrent relapses while receiving methotrexate or concerns regarding compliance [24].

4.3 Severe or diffuse forms of granulomatosis with polyangiitis

Both rituximab and cyclophosphamide, in combination with glucocorticoids, have been used for remission induction in GPA [24]. Corticosteroids with cyclophosphamide have always represented the gold standard in the treatment of diffuse forms of GPA. Cyclophosphamide can be administrated per os (2mg/kg/day) or by intravenous pulses (15mg/kgevery 2 weeks for the first 3 pulses then every 3 weeks) for an initial duration of 3 to 6 months. According to the studies, they have comparable results in terms of efficiency and average survival. However, due to the high cumulative dose of the oral route, this modality is associated with a high risk of infectious events [25, 26]. Rituximab or anti-CD20 is now preferred over cyclophosphamide for many reasons. Its efficiency in inducing remission has been proven by numerous studies, especially for relapsed diffuse forms [22, 27, 28]. It is a better-tolerated treatment and is considered less toxic than cyclophosphamide. It has lower risks of malignancy and/or infertility. Also, the risk of infectious complications is almost the same between these two drugs [29]. Rituximab has been approved for use in GPA as a weekly infusion of 375 mg/m2 for 4 consecutive weeks or as two 1-gram infusions spaced two weeks apart. Currently, it is prescribed for relapsed patients, those of childbearing age and/or those who have already received high cumulative doses of cyclophosphamide. A duration of 3 months may be required to achieve maximum therapeutic benefit.

As in all AAVs and by extrapolation to their efficiency in Goodpasture's syndrome, plasma exchange is indicated in severe forms of GPA with alveolar hemorrhage and/or glomerulonephritis. The MEPEX study showed their efficacy in patients with severe renal impairment (creatinine level over 500 umol/l), but this action is not maintained over the long term [30]. The benefit was most pronounced in patients with the highest risk of end-stage renal disease [24]. Polyvalent immunoglobulins are recommended for relapsing or severe disease. The total dose of infusions is 2 g/kg over 2 or 5 days.

4.4 Remission maintenance therapy

To reduce its iatrogenicity, gradual tapering of corticosteroids is preferable after inducing remission.

- Remission maintenance treatments for non-severe or limited forms of GPA are based on the same immunosuppressant used in the induction phase (methotrexate, MMF) [22]. Methotrexate should be taken for a long-term period (several years). According to the NORAM study, stopping methotrexate at one year of progression increases the risk of relapse of GPA [23]. For diffuse forms of GPA, methotrexate and azathioprine represented the conventional remission maintenance drugs in the last years. The WEGENT study concluded that they have comparable results in terms of efficiency, safety and relapse frequency [31]. Rituximab is mentioned in the latest European EULAR/ERA-EDTA guidelines as a remission maintenance drug. Several prospective and retrospective studies have compared rituximab with other molecules such as azathioprine. The results of these studies were in favor of a greater reduction in the relapse rate of GPA by rituximab [22]. Therefore, rituximab is now favored and highly recommended over methotrexate or azathioprine for maintaining remission of severe GPA, but cost and other factors may limit rituximab use [24]. Upon remission of GPA, this biomedicine is started within 1 month of the last cyclophosphamide infusion or 4 to 6 months after the start of rituximab induction therapy. It is administered in 5 infusions of 500 mg over 18 months (at D1 and D15 then every 6 months for 18 months) (FDA-approved) [22].

5. Treatment of eosinophilic granulomatosis with polyangiitis

5.1 Conventional therapeutic regimen

Like other AAV, corticosteroids are the treatment's cornerstone for GEPA. Depending on the severity of the presentation, high-dose corticosteroids are oftenly initiated with pulses of methylprednisolone (15 mg/kg). It is recommended for a minimum period of 4 weeks followed by a taper. This helps to control asthma, general signs and hypereosinophilia [32]. Corticosteroids are prescribed alone or combined with an immunosuppressant after evaluation of the clinical presentation by the FFS.

- If the FFS is equal to 0: These patients have no poor prognostic factors. Corticosteroids are sufficient to achieve remission in more than 70% of cases [32]. Cyclophosphamide is used in case of relapse or resistance to corticosteroids [33]. Survival rates in this group are important even in case of relapse.

- If the FFS is equal to or more than 1: Intravenous pulse cyclophosphamide should be combined. Treatment strategy recommends 6 pulses in less than 4 months (15 mg/kg every two weeks for three doses and then every three weeks for three doses). For remission maintenance, azathioprine at a dose of 2 mg/kg/day or methotrexate at a dose of 0.3 mg/Kg/week will be used for 12 to 18 months depending on the evolution [34].

5.2 Therapeutic alternatives

There have been very few randomized controlled trials conducted to date in EGPA. Rituximab is not yet validated as an alternative to cyclophosphamide in GEPA. Due to the rarity of this disease compared to other AAV, a small number of therapeutic trials have been reported in the literature with conflicting results. Some studies confirm the efficiency of this biomedicine especially in case of relapse [35–38] and particularly in patients with a positive vasculitis/anti-MPO profile [39]. Nevertheless, in addition to infectious complications, rituximab has been incriminated in the occurrence of severe bronchospasm secondary to a hypersensitivity reaction [39].

Recently, interleukin-5 inhibitors have been introduced into the GEPA therapeutic regimen. Mepolizumab is a humanized monoclonal antibody against interleukin-5. It has been approved for use in severe eosinophilic asthma. In refractory forms of GEPA, it was effective in remission induction and maintenance due to its immunosuppressive properties [40, 41]. A recent international randomized, controlled and double-blind study compared the effect of mepolizumab versus placebo in refractory GEPA treated with corticosteroids combined or not with immunosuppressive treatment. Long-term remission of GEPA was noted in the group using mepolizumab [42].

Anti-IgE drugs such as omalizumab have been used during severe allergic asthma. For GEPA, the results of the use of this biomedicine are variable and contradictory. As previously described, omalizumab has been incriminated as an unmasking factor for underlying vasculitis [43]. Other studies suggest its efficacy during GEPA especially for pulmonary relapses but also as a cortisone-sparing agent [44, 45]. In conclusion, further data are needed before omalizumab can be recommended or contraindicated in the treatment of GEPA [36].

6. Treatment of microscopic polyangiitis

Management of MPA is based on remission induction therapy and remission maintenance therapy. For non-renal forms with an FFS equal to zero, corticosteroids are used alone as a first-line treatment to induce remission. An immunosuppressant will be associated in case of non-response, relapse or dependence on corticosteroids but also in case of extension to a systemic form with involvement of other organs (cardiac, renal, CNS ...). However, high-dose corticosteroids associated with rituximab or cyclophosphamide are recommended for severe forms of MPA with a life-threatening outcome [22]. Azathioprine and methotrexate have been validated as remission maintenance treatments [31]. By extrapolation of their efficacy in good pasture's syndrome, plasma exchange is indicated in fulminant forms of MPA with severe renal involvement and/or alveolar hemorrhage. Currently, rituximab is also recommended for remission induction in case of refractory disease [28].

7. Associated treatments in ANCA-associated vasculitis

Management of AAV includes other therapeutic measures such as local and/ or surgical treatment of ENT manifestations in GPA and EGPA (nasal irrigations,

Type of vasculitis	Phase of treatment	Form of vasculitis	Recommendation/ statement	Level of evidence	Associated treatment
GPA/MPA	Remission induction therapy	Active non-severe/limited form of GPA	High dose of GCs + MTX (over CYC, RTX, AZA or MMF)	Very low to moderate	-Cotrimoxazole -Local or surgical treatment of ENT manifestations -Kinesitherapy and symptomatic treatments for neuropathic manifestations
		Active severe form of GPA/ MPA	High dose of GCs + RTX (over CYC)		
	Remission maintenance therapy	Non-severe/ limited form of GPA	GCs + MTX, AZA or MMF (continue the same medication)	–	
		severe form of GPA/MPA	Patients whose disease has entered remission after treatment with CYC or RTX: GCs + RTX (over MTX or AZA	Very low to moderate	
EGPA	Remission induction therapy	Active non-severe form of EGPA	GCs alone or with MEP (over MTX, AZA or MMF)	Very low to low	
		Active severe form of EGPA	High dose of GCs + either CYC or RTX (over MEP)	Very low	
	Remission maintenance therapy	Non-severe limited form of EGPA	CGs	–	
		severe form of EGPA	Patients whose disease has entered remission after treatment with CYC: GCs + MTX, AZA or MMF (over RTX or MEP)	Very low	

GPA: granulomatosis with polyangiitis, MPA: microscopic polyangiitis, EGPA: eosinophilic granulomatosis with polyangiitis, GCs: glucocorticoids MTX: methotrexate, AZA: azathioprine, MMF: mycophenolate mofetil, CYC: cyclophosphamide, MEP: mepolizumab, ENT: ear nose throat.

Table 4.
Recommendations/statements for the management of ANCA vasculitis [24].

nebulizations, polyposis resection ...), kinesitherapy and symptomatic treatments for neuropathic symptoms and hemodialysis in end-stage renal disease. In addition, complications related to the long-term use of corticosteroids should be managed (hypertension, diabetes ...) [28].

Cotrimoxazole (trimethoprim/sulfamethoxazole) is highly recommended in AAV and should be discussed in case of lymphopenia. Especially in GPA, it prevents from pneumocystis and has a role in remission maintenance of this vasculitis (**Table 4**).

8. Conclusion

Significant advancements in pathogenic knowledge helped to improve the management and the prognosis of patients suffering from AAV. This group of rare systemic vasculitis has now earlier remissions and lower relapse rates but needs urgent and aggressive treatment based on corticosteroids and immunosuppressant agents most of the time. Nowadays, rituximab has gained popularity because of his efficiency and less toxic properties. It is now preferred in severe cases of GPA and MPA. It was even more potent than cyclophosphamide in relapsing forms of the diseases. Our understanding of the pathogenesis continues to expand, and targeting specific pathogenic pathways is needed to improve the outcome.

Author details

Yosra Bouattour, Mouna Snoussi* and Zouhir Bahloul
Department of Internal Medicine, Hedi Chaker Hospital, Medical School of Sfax, Tunisia

*Address all correspondence to: mounasnoussi23@gmail.com

IntechOpen

© 2023 The Author(s). Licensee IntechOpen. This chapter is distributed under the terms of the Creative Commons Attribution License (http://creativecommons.org/licenses/by/3.0), which permits unrestricted use, distribution, and reproduction in any medium, provided the original work is properly cited.

References

[1] Meddeb Z, Larbi T, El Ouni A, Toujani S, Abdelkafi C, Hamzaoui S, et al. ANCA-associated vasculitis: About a Tunisian cohort. Review Internal Medicine. 2017;**38**:A116-A117

[2] Cohen Tervaert JW. Trimethoprim-sulfamethoxazole and antineutrophil cytoplasmic antibodies-associated vasculitis. Current Opinion in Rheumatology. 2018;**30**(4):388-394

[3] The European Vasculitis Study Group. French Vasculitis Study Group. Disponible en: http:// www.vascularites.org/index.php

[4] Ilva F, Cisternas M. Vasculitis asociadas a anticuerpos anti-citoplasma de neutrófilos: avances en patogenia y tratamiento [anti-neutrophil cytoplasmic antibody (ANCA)-associated vasculitis: Advances in pathogenesis and treatment]. Revista Médica de Chile. 2013;**141**(6):765-773

[5] Geetha D, Jefferson JA. ANCA-associated Vasculitis: Core curriculum 2020. American Journal of Kidney Diseases. 2020;**75**(1):124-137

[6] Lionaki S, Blyth ER, Hogan SL, et al. Classification of antineutrophil cytoplasmic autoantibody vasculitides: The role of antineutrophil cytoplasmic autoantibody specificity for myeloperoxidase or proteinase 3 in disease recognition and prognosis. Arthritis and Rheumatism. 2012;**64**(10):3452-3462

[7] Mouthon L, Millet A, Regent A, Pederzoli-Ribeil M, Witko-Sarsat V. Pathophysiology of ANCA-positive vasculitides. Presse Médicale. 2012;**41**(10):996-1003

[8] Li W, Huang H, Cai M, Yuan T, Sheng Y. Antineutrophil cytoplasmic antibody-associated Vasculitis update: Genetic pathogenesis. Frontiers in Immunology. 2021;**26**:624848

[9] Watts RA, Mahr A, Mohammad AJ, Gatenby P, Basu N, Flores-Suarez LF. Classification, epidemiology and clinical subgrouping of antineutrophil cytoplasmic antibody (ANCA)-associated vasculitis. Nephrology Dialysis Transplantation. 2015;**30**(suppl_1): i14-i22

[10] Watts RA, Lane SE, Scott DG, Koldingsnes W, Nossent H, Gonzalez-Gay MA, et al. Epidemiology of vasculitis in Europe. Annals of the Rheumatic Diseases. 2001;**60**(12):1156-1157

[11] de Guevara DL, Cerda F, Carreño MA, Piottante A, Bitar P. Update in the study of granulomatosis with polyangiitis (Wegener's granulomatosis). Revista Chilena de Radiologia. 2019;**25**(1):26-34

[12] Salah RB, Frikha F, Snoussi M, Abderrahmen M, Hentati Y, Mnif Z, et al. Limited form of Wegener's granulomatosis in a patient with Crohn's disease. A case report. The. Turkish Journal of Gastroenterology. 2014;**25**(Suppl.-1):191-195

[13] Robson JC, Grayson P, Ponte C, Suppiah R, Craven A, Judge A, et al. 2022 American College of Rheumatology/ European Alliance of associations for rheumatology classification criteria for granulomatosis with polyangiitis. Arthritis and Rheumatology. 2022;*74*(3):393-399

[14] Watts RA, Lane S, Scott DGI. What is known about the epidemiology of the vasculitides? Best Practice

Research Clinical Rheumatology. 2005;**19**(2):191-207

[15] Zwerina J, Eger G, Englbrecht M, Manger B, Schett G. Churg–Strauss syndrome in childhood: A systematic literature review and clinical comparison with adult patients. Seminars in Arthritis and Rheumatism. 2009;**39**:108-115

[16] Piram M, Maldini C, Mahr A. Effect of race/ethnicity on risk, presentation and course of connective tissue diseases and primary systemic vasculitides. Current Opinion in Rheumatology. 2012;**24**:193-200

[17] Masi AT, Hunder GG, Lie JT, Michel BA, Bloch DA, Arend WP, et al. The American College of Rheumatology criteria for the classification of Churg–Strauss syndrome (allergic granulomatosis and angiitis). Arthritis & Rheumatology. 1990;**33**:1094-1100

[18] Pagnoux C, Guilpain P, Guillevin L. Churg–Strauss syndrome. Current Opinion in Rheumatology. 2007;**19**:25-32

[19] Pagnoux C, Guilpain P, Guillevin L. Polyangéite microscopique. Presse Médicale. 2007;**36**(5):895-901

[20] Puéchal X, Pagnoux C, Baron G, Quémeneur T, Néel A, Agard C, et al. Adding azathioprine to remission-induction glucocorticoids for eosinophilic granulomatosis with polyangiitis (Churg-Strauss), microscopic polyangiitis, or polyarteritis nodosa without poor prognosis factors: A randomized, controlled trial. Arthritis. Rheumatology. 2017;**69**(11):2175-2186

[21] Guillevin L, Pagnoux C, Seror R, Mahr A, Mouthon L, Toumelin PL. French Vasculitis Study Group (FVSG). The Five-Factor Score revisited: assessment of prognoses of systemic necrotizing vasculitides based on the French Vasculitis Study Group (FVSG) cohort. Medicine (Baltimore). Jan 2011;**90**(1)

[22] Makhzoum J-P, Pagnoux C. Actualités thérapeutiques de la granulomatose avec polyangéite (Wegener) et de la polyangéite microscopique. Review in Rheumatic Monograph. 2017;**84**(3):242-248

[23] De Groot K, Rasmussen N, Bacon PA, Tervaert JWC, Feighery C, Gregorini G, et al. Randomized trial of cyclophosphamide versus methotrexate for induction of remission in early systemic antineutrophil cytoplasmic antibody-associated vasculitis. Arthritis Rheumatology. 2005;**52**(8):2461-2469

[24] Chung SA, Langford CA, Maz M, Abril A, Gorelik M, Guyatt G, et al. 2021 American College of Rheumatology/ Vasculitis Foundation guideline for the Management of Antineutrophil Cytoplasmic Antibody-Associated Vasculitis. Arthritis & Rhematology. 2021;**73**(8):1366-1383

[25] de Groot K, Adu D, Savage CO, EUVAS (European vasculitis study group). The value of pulse cyclophosphamide in ANCA-associated vasculitis: meta-analysis and critical review. Nephrology Dialysis Transplantation Off Publ Eur Dial Transpl Assoc. 2001;**16**(10):2018-2027

[26] Harper L, Morgan MD, Walsh M, Hoglund P, Westman K, Flossmann O, et al. Pulse versus daily oral cyclophosphamide for induction of remission in ANCA-associated vasculitis: Long-term follow-up. Annals of Rheumatic Diseases. 2012;**71**(6):955-960

[27] Keogh KA, Wylam ME, Stone JH, Specks U. Induction of remission by B lymphocyte depletion in eleven

patients with refractory antineutrophil cytoplasmic antibody-associated vasculitis. Arthritis Rheumatic. 2005;**52**(1):262-268

[28] Jones RB, Ferraro AJ, Chaudhry AN, Brogan P, Salama AD, Smith KGC, et al. A multicenter survey of rituximab therapy for refractory antineutrophil cytoplasmic antibody-associated vasculitis. Arthritis Rheumatic. 2009;**60**(7):2156-2168

[29] Stone JH, Merkel PA, Spiera R, Seo P, Langford CA, Hoffman GS, et al. Rituximab versus cyclophosphamide for ANCA-associated Vasculitis. The New England Journal of Medicine. 2010;**363**(3):221-232

[30] Jayne DRW, Gaskin G, Rasmussen N, Abramowicz D, Ferrario F, Guillevin L, et al. Randomized trial of plasma exchange or high-dosage methylprednisolone as adjunctive therapy for severe renal vasculitis. Journal of American Society Nephrology JASN. 2007;**18**(7):2180-2188

[31] Long-Term Outcomes Among Participants in the WEGENT Trial of Remission. Maintenance Therapy for Granulomatosis With Polyangiitis (Wegener's) or Microscopique Polyangiitis. Arthritis Rheumatology. 2016;**68**(3):690-701

[32] Charles P, Terrier B, Perrodeau É, Cohen P, Faguer S, Huart A, et al. Comparison of individually tailored versus fixed-schedule rituximab regimen to maintain ANCA-associated vasculitis remission: Results of a multicentre, randomised controlled, phase III trial (MAINRITSAN2). Annals of Rheumatic Diseases. 2018;**77**(8):1143-1149

[33] La GL. granulomatose éosinophilique avec polyangéite (syndrome de Churg et Strauss). Presse Médicale. 2012;**41**(10):1004-1013

[34] Ribi C, Cohen P, Pagnoux C, Mahr A, Arène J-P, Lauque D, et al. Treatment of Churg-Strauss syndrome without poor-prognosis factors: A multicenter, prospective, randomized, open-label study of seventy-two patients. Arthritis Rheumatic. 2008;**58**(2):586-594

[35] Moosig F, Holle J. Aktuelle Therapie der eosinophilen Granulomatose mit polyangiitis (Churg-Strauss-Syndrom). Z Für Rheumatol. 2019;**78**:333-338

[36] Raffray L, Guillevin L. Updates for the treatment of EGPA. Presse Med. 2020;**49**(3):104036

[37] Fanouriakis A, Kougkas N, Vassilopoulos D, Fragouli E, Repa A, Sidiropoulos P. Rituximab for eosinophilic granulomatosis with polyangiitis with severe vasculitic neuropathy: Case report and review of current clinical evidence. Seminars in Arthritis Rheumatology. 2015;**45**(1):60-66

[38] Charles P, Bienvenu B, Bonnotte B, Gobert P, Godmer P, Hachulla É, et al. Rituximab: Recommendations of the French Vasculitis study group (FVSG) for induction and maintenance treatments of adult, antineutrophil cytoplasm antibody-associated necrotizing vasculitides. Presse Médicale. 2013;**42**(10):1317-1330

[39] Bouldouyre M-A, Cohen P, Guillevin L. Severe bronchospasm associated with rituximab for refractory Churg-Strauss syndrome. Annals of the Rheumatic Diseases. 2009;**68**(4):606-606

[40] Kim S, Marigowda G, Oren E, Israel E, Wechsler ME. Mepolizumab as a steroid-sparing treatment option in patients with Churg-Strauss syndrome. Journal of Allergy Clinical Immunology. 2010;**125**(6):1336-1343

[41] Moosig F, Gross WL, Herrmann K, Bremer JP, Hellmich B. Targeting Interleukin-5 in Refractory and Relapsing Churg–Strauss Syndrome. Annals of Internal Medicine. 2011;**155**(5):341

[42] Wechsler ME, Akuthota P, Jayne D, Khoury P, Klion A, Langford CA, et al. Mepolizumab or placebo for eosinophilic granulomatosis with polyangiitis. The New England Journal of Medicine. 2017;**376**(20):1921-1932

[43] Bekçibaşı M, Barutçu S, Çelen MK, Dayan S, Hoşoğlu S. Churg-Strauss syndrome occurring during omalizumab treatment. European Journal of Rheumatology. 2015;**2**(3):129-130

[44] Naudion P, Méaux-Ruault N, Gil H, Humbert S, Bouiller K, Magy-Bertrand N. Le traitement de la granulomatose éosinophilique avec polyangéite réfractaire par omalizumab : à propos de 4 cas. Rev Médecine Interne. déc. 2016;**37**:A263

[45] Koukoulaki M. Rituximab in Churg-Strauss syndrome. Annals of Rheumatic Diseases. 2006;**65**(4):557-559

Section 5

Post-COVID-19 Pericardial Diseases

Chapter 6

The Evaluation of Myocarditis in the Post-Covid-19 Era: Pearls and Perils for the Clinician

Daniel Zinkovsky and Michael R. Sood

Abstract

Coronavirus disease 2019 (COVID-19), which is caused by the Severe Acute Respiratory Syndrome Coronavirus 2 (SARS-CoV-2), continues to remain a global threat since declared a pandemic by the World Health Organization in March 2020. While primarily a respiratory disease, its clinical manifestations vary widely ranging from asymptomatic infection to multi-organ failure and death. As more research becomes available, cardiovascular involvement including acute coronary syndrome, heart failure, arrhythmias, thromboembolism, myocarditis and pericarditis have been reported in both the acute infectious stage as well as the post-symptomatic period. Myocarditis is an inflammatory disease of the myocardium that can result from infectious or non-infectious causes including autoimmunity, drug and toxin exposures. This chapter discusses the incidence, pathology, diagnostic modalities, and the management of myocarditis with a special focus on the essential role of a comprehensive approach, while utilizing advanced cardiac imaging for the assessment of myocarditis in the post COVID-19 era.

Keywords: cardiac MRI, CMR, COVID-19, Dallas criteria, endomyocardial biopsy, Lake Louise criteria, myocarditis, SARS-CoV-2 mRNA vaccine

1. Introduction

As of October 2022, the COVID-19 pandemic has been responsible for over 1 million deaths in the United States and over 6.5 million deaths globally [1, 2]. Its clinical manifestations range from asymptomatic to a mild, self-limited infection, to severe multi-organ failure and/or death. Due to the wide spectrum of illness and organ involvement as well as the diversity of cardiovascular manifestations and methods for its diagnosis, myocarditis can pose a particular challenge to clinicians.

Myocarditis is an inflammatory disease of the myocardium that can weaken the efficiency of the heart to pump blood or interfere with its conduction system. Most commonly, it occurs as a result from viral infection or autoimmune activation, toxins, drugs, or vaccine exposure. The diagnosis ranges widely and can be made based on history and various clinical aspects or via biopsy, which relies on an established criteria including histologic and immunohistochemical evidence. In 1986, the proposed

IntechOpen

Dallas criteria established histopathological classifications to aid in the diagnosis of myocarditis requiring evidence of an inflammatory infiltrate with or without associated myocyte necrosis/fibrosis unrelated to ischemia [3]. Endomyocardial biopsy has remained the gold standard for diagnosis, despite recent advances in imaging technologies. However, postmortem analysis has revealed many limitations, stemming from challenges in specimens and sampling errors, in addition to variation in expert interpretation [4]. Furthermore, numerous studies have shown that a virus may be present in the myocardium in a replicative or non-replicative form in the absence of inflammation sufficient to meet the Dallas criteria [5, 6].

More commonly in clinical practice, a patient's clinical symptoms, laboratory tests and imaging studies—including the use of cardiac magnetic resonance imaging (CMR)—is not only sufficient to establish a diagnosis but represents a non-invasive alternative to biopsy. CMR can detect early myocardial tissue response such as edema, hyperemia, and necrosis, as well as late consequences such as myocardial fibrosis and provide enhanced information that can be utilized in prognostication and clinical decision making [7].

2. Etiology/pathogenesis

The global incidence of myocarditis in 2017 was 3,071,000 cases, a 59.6% increase from 1990 according to data from the Global Burden of Disease Study 2017 [8]. However, the exact incidence is difficult to determine as myocarditis has a variable clinical presentation mimicking other conditions and can coexist with other cardiac or systemic diseases. Furthermore, there is limited availability of advanced cardiac imaging or endomyocardial biopsy, which can also contribute to confirming its diagnosis. Thus, the actual cases of myocarditis are believed to be significantly underestimated [9].

2.1 Infectious

Infectious causes remain the most frequent causes of myocarditis globally with viral etiology more common in the developed countries of North America and Europe, while bacterial, protozoal, fungal, and other rare pathogens are responsible for most cases in the developing countries of Africa, Asia, and South America [10]. A comprehensive list of currently identified infectious causes of myocarditis can be found in **Table 1**.

Bacterial myocarditis is rare, but the most common cause is *Staphylococcus aureus* and Streptococcal species [16]. The prevalence is difficult to determine with few studies published reporting 0.2–1.5% from cardiac biopsy samples post-mortem [17]. Furthermore, its prevalence has been shown to be more common in the setting of sepsis with or without concomitant endocarditis. The pathogenesis typically involves direct bacterial invasion into cardiac myocytes or by pathogenic toxins (common with clostridium or diphtheria). Cardiac dysfunction of either the left or right ventricle subsequently develops from severe sepsis (mediated by increased circulating cytokines), myocardial inflammation/necrosis, direct action from toxins and in the later stages, ventricular remodeling.

Viral myocarditis is by far the most common etiology with an incidence in the range of 10–22 per 100,000 individuals [18]. The pathogenesis follows a similar course of other pathogens that involve direct myocardial invasion with three distinct

Viral	Adenoviruses, HBV, HCV, HH6, HSV 1 and 2, Chikungunya virus, SARS COV-2, Coxsackie virus, Dengue virus HIV, CMV, EBV, Influenza, Parvovirus B19, Measles virus, Mumps virus, Polioviruses, Rabies virus, Respiratory syncytial virus, Rubella virus, Varicella-Zoster virus, Variola virus, Vaccinia virus, Yellow fever virus
Bacterial	Brucella, Chlamydia, Clostidrium, Corynebacterium diphtheria, Haemophilus influenzae, Gonococcus, Legionella spp, Meningococcus, Mycobacteria, Mycoplasma pneumoniae, Pneumococcus, Salmonella, Staphylococcus, Streptococci, Vibrio cholera
Protozoa	Entamoeba histolytica, Leishmania, Plasmodium falciparum, Trypanosoma cruzi, Toxoplasma gondii
Spirochete	Borrelia burgdorferi, Leptospira, Treponema pallidum
Fungal	Actinomyces, Aspergillus, Blastomyces, Candida, Coccidioides, Cryptococcus, Histoplasma, Mucormycoses, Nocardia, Sporothrix schenckii
Parasites/Rickettsia	Echinococcus granulosus, Schistosoma, Taenia solium, Toxocara canis, Trichinella spiralis, Coxiella burnetii, Rickettsia rickettsii

Abbreviations: CMV—Cytomegalovirus; EBV—Epstein-Barr virus; HBV—Hepatitis B virus; HCV—Hepatitis C virus; HH6—human herpesvirus 6; HIV—human immunodeficiency virus; HSV—Herpes Simplex virus

Table 1.
Infectious causes of myocarditis [11–15].

phases: acute, subacute, and chronic. Each phase is characterized by a distinct process with variable transitional periods. In phase 1 (acute), the virus gains access into the target organ tissue and triggers an immune response. This may progress into phase 2 (subacute), an autoimmune phase involving autoreactive T-cells, cytokines, and cross-reacting antibodies predominant after the full or partial resolution of the initial infection. Finally, in phase 3 (chronic), there is progressive remodeling often from autoimmune injury to the myocardium resulting in a persistent or often dilated cardiomyopathy [18, 19].

The **acute phase** includes the first days following infection where viral replication occurs within the heart and other organs. Viral entry is largely facilitated by specific receptors that vary based on the pathogen. For instance, Measles virus entry depends on the major reovirus receptor JAM-A, SARS-CoV-2 utilizes the spike protein to bind the ACE2 receptor and in Group B coxsackieviruses (CVB) viral entry is mediated via two host receptors, decay-accelerating factor (DAF) and coxsackievirus-adeno-virus receptor (CAR). In the case of coxsackievirus, these receptors are expressed in cardiac myocytes and pancreatic cells. Animal models have demonstrated the important role they play in so much that targeted deletion of these receptors is protective against CVB-induced pancreatitis and myocarditis [20]. Following initial viral entry, the virus causes cell lysis and spreads infection to adjacent cells through release of packaged virions. The cardiomyocyte injury triggers an innate immune response increasing the levels of cytokines and infiltration of immune cells into the damaged tissue (seen in **Figure 1**).

Approximately 1 week following infection, the **subacute**, autoimmune phase develops in response to the immune dysregulation caused by myocyte injury via molecular mimicry of the viral antigens to host cardiac proteins [22]. It should be noted that acute reduction in LV function along with hemodynamic compromise can occur during acute and subacute phases. The constant activation of T cells, increased levels of cytokines including tumor necrosis factor-α (TNF-α), interleukin (IL)-1,

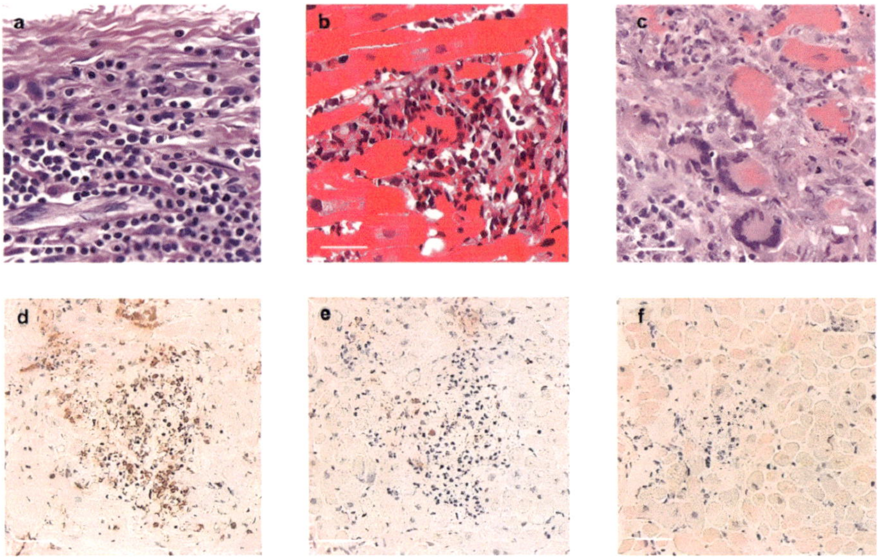

Figure 1.
Fulminant Myocarditis (FM) pathological phenotypes. a–c representative HE staining of EMB samples of FM patients showed lymphocyte FM (a), eosinophilic FM (b), and giant cell FM (c). d–f IHC staining showed massive T lymphocyte (CD45RO) infiltrated into myocardium (d). Macrophage (CD68) can also be observed (e). Few B lymphocytes (CD20) can be seen in EMB samples (f). From [21]. Copyright © Hang et al. Distributed under the terms of the Creative Commons Attribution 4.0 International License.

and IL-6, may lead to persistent and recurrent myocardial damage causing further impairment of the heart's contractile function and progressive remodeling, which is seen in the chronic phase of the disease.

In the final, **chronic phase** of the disease, the cumulative effect of the virus either through direct cytotoxic or subsequent autoimmune damage initiates a process of myocardial remodeling that can lead to dilated cardiomyopathy. In most cases by the chronic stage, the virus has been cleared and inflammation subsided, but in some cases the chronic phase is associated with a persistent viral infection and ongoing autoimmune responses. In myocarditis patients with chronic symptoms and inflammation, parvovirus B19 (PVB19) and human herpesvirus 6 (HHV6) genomes predominate in EMB samples with approximately 30% of patients having multiple viral infections [23].

2.2 Drug/toxin induced

Toxic drug-induced myocarditis is inflammation of the myocardium from drugs used as part of medical treatment or recreation. Damage is often by direct cytotoxic effect and/or immune-mediated but in many cases the concomitant mechanisms are poorly understood. **Table 2** lists many of the currently identified drugs/toxins reported to induce myocarditis with a recent analysis of World Health Organization pharmacovigilance database recognizing five distinct categories of drugs: antipsychotics, cytotoxic drugs, immunotherapies, vaccines, and salicylates [11–15, 24–30]. Although patients are not routinely screened, they share many distinct similarities in presentation and clinicians should have heightened awareness to such etiologies. Cardiac injury can be either acute or progressive but frequently irreversible (even if

Antipsychotics	Phenothiazines, Tricyclic antidepressants, Lithium, Clozapine
Vaccines	Smallpox, Influenza, Anthrax, DTPP, HepA/HepB, Meningococcal, COVID-19
Immunotherapy (including Immune Checkpoint inhibitors)	Ipilimumab, Nivolumab, Pembrolizumab, Atezolizumab, Durvalumab, Avelumab, Cemiplimab
Cytotoxic	5-Fluorouracil, Anthracyclines, Cyclophosphamide
Salicylate	Mesalazine, Sulfasalazine
Drugs of abuse	Amphetamines, Cocaine, Alcohol, ephedrine
Cardiac medications	Dobutamine, Epinephrine, Norepinephrine, Dopamine

Table 2.
Drugs/toxins known to cause toxic myocarditis [11–15, 24–32].

recognized early in its course), manifesting with new onset arrhythmias, a bundle branch block and in its end stage as an idiopathic dilated cardiomyopathy. Like other causes, resulting inflammation and myocyte destruction gives way to fibrous tissue replacement. In the case of antipsychotics such as clozapine, it is believed that a type 1 hypersensitivity reaction to clozapine itself or its cardiotoxic metabolite triggers a rise in inflammatory mediators [31].

Immune checkpoint inhibitors (ICI) which enhance T-cell mediated immune responses for the treatment of a variety of malignancies are effective but are associated with either fulminant or insidious myocarditis. While the incidence of myocarditis with these agents is rare, ranging from 0.27% to 1.14%, it is associated with a high mortality rate of 40–50% in those affected [32]. The risk was greatest with the combination therapy utilizing anti-cytotoxic T-lymphocyte associated protein 4 (anti-CTLA-4) and anti-programmed cell death 1 (anti-PD 1) agents. ICI-associated myocarditis is unique histologically demonstrating myocardial infiltration of T lymphocytes and macrophages with direct involvement of the conduction system leading to more observed arrhythmias upon presentation with a lower incidence of heart failure when compared to other forms of myocarditis such as viral and autoimmune in which inflammation ultimately leads to dilated cardiomyopathy [30].

Hypersensitivity reactions with eosinophilic myocarditis are associated with both antipsychotic agents and salicylates while ICIs are associated with lymphocytic myocarditis (**Figure 1**). Direct cardiac cytotoxicity, apoptosis and free radical oxidative damage are predominant features of cytotoxic antineoplastic agents. Vaccine associated myocarditis, on the other hand, such as seen with smallpox is primarily an autoimmune mediated response from the vaccine's ability to mimic myocardial antigens [11].

2.3 Autoimmune

While immune activation has a prominent role in the pathophysiology of myocarditis secondary to infectious or selected drug-induced process as previously described, systemic immune-mediated diseases that include systemic lupus erythematosus (SLE), antiphospholipid syndrome (APS), vasculitis (such as eosinophilic granulomatosis and polyangiitis (EGPA)), sarcoidosis and even organ-based immune mediated diseases such as chronic inflammatory bowel diseases may be associated with myocarditis [33].

Eosinophilic myocarditis can be seen with autoimmune diseases (SLE, EGPA, inflammatory bowel disease), hypersensitivity to select medications (antibiotics, sulfa-drugs, anticonvulsants, diuretics), hematologic nonmyeloid malignancies (lymphoma, acute myeloid leukemia, acute lymphoblastic leukemia) as well as infectious (parasitic, fungal, HIV) causes [34]. It should be suspected in patients with peripheral blood eosinophilia >1.5G/L and symptoms of acute coronary syndrome or heart failure but without obstructive coronary disease. Additional clues may include rash or elevated liver function tests. Rate of death or cardiac transplantation with a fulminant presentation of eosinophilic myocarditis can exceed 26% in only 60 days [35]. A resulting cardiomyopathy proceeds along three stages progressing from (1) infiltration of myocardium by eosinophils, (2) thrombosis driven largely by endomyocardial damage and alteration of systemic coagulation via enhanced tissue factor expression and impaired thrombomodulin, (3) biventricular *endomyocardial* scarring and fibrosis from activation of cardiac mast cells to the released eosinophilic granules [36].

Giant cell myocarditis (GCM) on the other hand, is associated with thymomas, inflammatory bowel disease, autoimmune disorders, drug hypersensitivity and is considered among the most fatal forms of myocarditis with studies indicating a rate of death or cardiac transplantation of approximately 70% [37]. In particular, giant-cell myocarditis has been shown to be histologically similar to cardiac sarcoidosis. A retrospective audit of 73 cases of GCM diagnosed in Finland since the late 1980s found that 60% of the original GCM diagnoses required conversion to cardiac sarcoidosis [38]. Myocardial necrosis and granulomas are present in both cardiac sarcoidosis and GCM although necrosis is typically more extensive in GCM where both eosinophils and lymphocytes are found in higher numbers, while granulomas are more common in cardiac sarcoidosis which has a greater extent of myocardial fibrosis [39]. This overlap is important to consider when the early diagnosis of GCM with calcineurin based immunosuppressive therapy can reduce the complications and mortality over cardiac sarcoidosis in which the mainstay of treatment consists of glucocorticoids.

Systemic lupus erythematosus (SLE) is another autoimmune disease commonly with cardiac and extracardiac involvement. Cardiac injury can occur from immunological injury, ischemia from accelerated atherosclerosis, as well as valvular disease from immunoglobulin and complement deposition. Although pericarditis is more common, lupus myocarditis occurs at a prevalence of 9% but is believed to have a higher prevalence in a subclinical form with 57% seen on autopsy [40]. Given the heterogeneous cardiac manifestations in systemic immune-mediated diseases, screening for autoimmune disease is recommended in patients with clinically suspected myocarditis for prompt diagnosis and appropriate management [41].

2.4 COVID-19/COVID vaccine

Recent studies estimate the incidence of cardiac injury ranging between 7 to 30% of patients with COVID-19 [33, 34]. This cardiac injury is believed to be multifactorial, caused by direct viral infection of the myocardium, complications from the widespread systemic inflammatory response, in addition to the prothrombotic changes including plaque rupture, demand ischemia or vasospasm [35]. The variability in symptoms and complications of SARS-CoV-2 infection has been presumed to be the result of the viral spike protein's utilization of its functional receptor, the angiotensin converting enzyme-2 (ACE-2), which has widespread expression on pulmonary alveolar cells, cardiac myocytes, gastrointestinal epithelial cells, and vascular endothelial cells [36]. Determining the true incidence of myocarditis is challenging, limited by the lack of endomyocardial biopsy in many presumed cases which would allow for histological confirmation or isolation of SARS-CoV2 virus in the myocardium.

In a meta-analysis of 31 case studies including 51 patients with suspected COVID-19 associated myocarditis, males were more commonly affected (69%) with a median age of 55 years (range 28–60 years) [37]. Another cohort single center study of 416 patients hospitalized with COVID-19 had an older median age of 64 years and balanced gender distribution with females affected at 50.7%. Of the total patients, 19.7% had cardiac injury, which tended to be older (median age 74), with more comorbidities (59% had hypertension), that commonly required noninvasive mechanical ventilation, had more complications (acute respiratory distress syndrome, acute kidney injury, electrolyte disturbances, coagulation disorders) and had a higher mortality than those without cardiac injury (51% vs. 4.5%) [38]. Numerous autopsy studies had demonstrated the widespread distribution of SARS-CoV-2 viral infiltration and replication in various body tissues including the respiratory tract, brain and cardiac myocytes [39, 40]. The virus can persist in these tissues without a concomitant inflammatory or immune mediated response.

Following widespread COVID-19 vaccination efforts specifically with the SARS-CoV-2 mRNA vaccines, myocarditis and myopericarditis cases were increasingly being reported in the literature. The estimated incidence ranges from 4 to 29.8 cases per million doses, most commonly seen in males aged $\leq$40 years following the second dose and presenting with symptoms on day 3 through 7 post-vaccination. The mechanism behind vaccine induced myopericarditis is believed to be caused in part by molecular mimicry of antibodies against SARS-CoV-2 spike protein and a self-antigen, increased IL-18-mediated immune responses and aberrant induction of apoptosis [41]. It is not associated with eosinophilia, thrombosis or mast cell activation.

3. Clinical presentation/diagnosis

Due to a varied clinical presentation and potential insidious processes of myocarditis, ranging from asymptomatic to congestive heart failure, hemodynamic compromise with shock or death, the diagnosis can be a challenge for the experienced clinician. The severity of clinical presentation can serve as a potential predictor of the prognosis with those exhibiting hemodynamic instability and or systolic dysfunction (LVEF < 50%) on admission suffering the highest risk of death or need of transplantation [42].

The most commonly presenting symptoms include fever, shortness of breath, cough, and chest pain (which can often overlap with pericarditis) or Myocardial Infarction with Non-obstructive Coronary Arteries (MINOCA) type syndrome, associated with elevated troponin on labs and regional wall motion abnormalities on echocardiogram. These patients tend to have generally good outcomes as opposed to other presentations of myocarditis that include heart failure (or acute cardiomyopathy), ventricular tachycardia, heart block or sudden death.

A patient with suspected myocarditis may present with a constellation of abnormal findings on laboratory, ECG, Echocardiogram and cardiac MRI. On ECG, many patients demonstrate non-specific ST segment and T wave changes that are present in addition to ventricular tachycardia or premature ventricular complexes. Elevated cardiac (Troponin, NT-pro-BNP) and inflammatory biomarkers (WBC, IL-6, CRP) are common as well as left ventricular dysfunction and hypokinesis on echocardiogram [37]. In the multicenter ITAMY study of 386 patients with acute myocarditis, most patients were young males (75% male, average age of 35), with preserved LVEF (62%) presenting with chest pain (95%), troponin elevation (100%, average peak 1.85 ng/ml), ECG abnormalities (96%), and wall motion abnormalities on echo (21%). An anteroseptal pattern on CMR was most associated with increased risk of major cardiac events (MACE) when compared to the inferolateral pattern which had the lowest risk of any LGE pattern [43]. Despite the gold standard diagnosis via myocardial biopsy, there is not one specific diagnostic criterion for the evaluation of myocarditis and advancements in cardiac imaging have led this evolution [44]. Therefore, a comprehensive evaluation is prudent and thus, we will discuss various imaging modalities further in this section.

3.1 Laboratory studies

To identify patients with suspected acute myocarditis, initial workup may involve laboratory tests for biomarkers of cardiac injury (troponin I, creatinine kinase-MB (CK-MB), Natriuretic Peptides (BNP or NT-proBNP)), inflammatory markers (C-reactive protein (CRP), erythrocyte sedimentation rate (ESR)), and differential white blood cell count (which can reveal eosinophilia) are routinely recommended. However, despite the availability of cardiac and inflammatory biomarkers, these may pose a challenge in the diagnosis of myocarditis as each of these markers, respectively, may be elevated in response to systemic illness (such as from tachycardic states, catecholamine excess, hypoxia driven myocardial stress and/or dysfunction), or other extra-cardiac organ dysfunction such as anemia or renal failure. Therefore, the utilization in surveillance of such biomarkers in relation to other clinical parameters (symptoms, physical examination, timing) and various imaging modalities, comprehensively, is recommended.

Troponin I has been shown to be highly specific (89%) but has limited sensitivity (34%) and superior to CK-MB in the diagnosis of myocarditis [45]. CK-MB elevations occur less frequently than troponin elevations in acute myocarditis. Plasma BNP, a cardiac neurohormone released in response to increased ventricular stress, is an important laboratory marker with a high positive predictive value for the diagnosis of heart failure. Like other biomarkers, it has been shown to be elevated in other cardiac etiologies such as acute coronary syndrome [46]. In acute myocarditis, patients with high baseline NT-proBNP had the highest rate of major adverse cardiac events both at 30 days and up to 3 years follow up, suggesting higher levels are predictors of poor outcomes [47]. Similarly, in the case of COVID-19, NT-proBNP is commonly elevated and high levels were significantly correlated to increased risk of death [48]. Inflammatory markers such as CRP are positive in 80–95% of cases of myocarditis in addition to ESR, in which persistent elevations could suggest an underlying autoimmune disorder [49].

Other less common serologic tests or virological tests can be considered to narrow the differential diagnosis in select patients presenting with myocarditis from infectious or autoimmune causes which include, HIV and Borrelia burgdorferi antibodies, polymerase chain reaction from samples of the respiratory tract (influenza and SARS-CoV-2), and autoantibodies (antinuclear antibodies) to name a few.

3.2 ECG

Myocarditis can present with a multitude of electrocardiographic (ECG) abnormalities across a spectrum of tachy- or bradyarrhythmia. Mechanisms for these

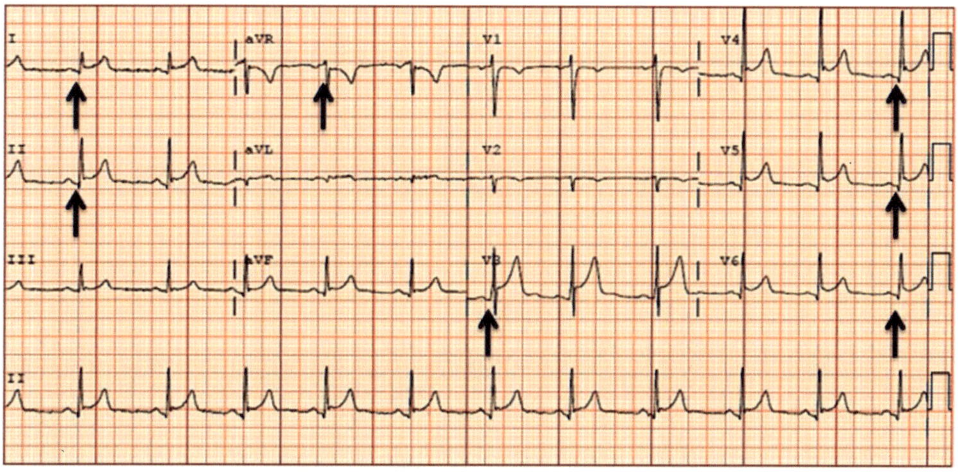

Figure 2.
12-lead electrocardiogram (ECG) in a 22-year-old male without any known cardiovascular conditions presenting 2 days after receiving first dose of COVID-19 vaccine (BNT162b2) showing diffuse PR segment depression and PR segment elevation in lead aVR (black arrows). From [50]˙ Copyright © Patel et al. 2021. Distributed under the terms of the Creative Commons Attribution 4.0 International License.

observed changes are believed to result from direct myocardial damage, high catecholamine states with elevated sympathetic or parasympathetic tone, and conditions of high interleukins or inflammatory-mediated myocardial damage. These conduction alterations may also be associated with concomitant structural abnormalities such as left or right ventricular chamber dilatation in various stages of myocarditis. Sinus tachycardia associated with nonspecific ST/T-wave changes are the most common ECG findings in myocarditis, while patterns of PR segment depressions in leads with ST segment elevation (STE), precordial and limb leads, or a PR segment elevation in aVR generally favors the diagnosis of pericarditis or peri-myocarditis (**Figure 2**). STE and T wave inversions (TWI) may be evident in various phases of myocarditis due to varying voltage difference in depolarization and repolarization exhibited between the epicardial and endocardial layers in the setting of myocarditis. Often this may overlap with STE mimicking that of ischemic injury pattern from obstructive coronary artery disease or pericardial involvement. Reports have also shown STE on presentation similar to that of an acute STE myocardial infarction without any proven obstructive coronary artery disease, and where the initial ECG findings and STE corresponded to areas of non-ischemic scar pattern seen later on CMR (**Figure 3**) [51]. The ECG features most associated with a poor prognosis in patients presenting with acute myocarditis are pathological Q waves, wide QRS complex, QRS/T angle ≥100°, prolonged QT interval, high-degree atrioventricular block and malignant ventricular tachyarrhythmia (Ventricular tachycardia (VT), ventricular fibrillation (VF), and torsades de pointes) [52].

In a study of 800 patients with COVID-19 at Mount Sinai Hospital, VT or VF contributed to 11% of the mortality [53]. Additionally, a small retrospective study of 275 patients presenting to the emergency department with COVID-19 found most ECGs were in normal sinus rhythm, with 10% of patients having atrial fibrillation/flutter, and another 40% with repolarization abnormalities including negative T waves in 21% of all abnormalities. The finding of an abnormal axis or left bundle branch block was significantly associated with in-hospital mortality [54]. In a larger observational

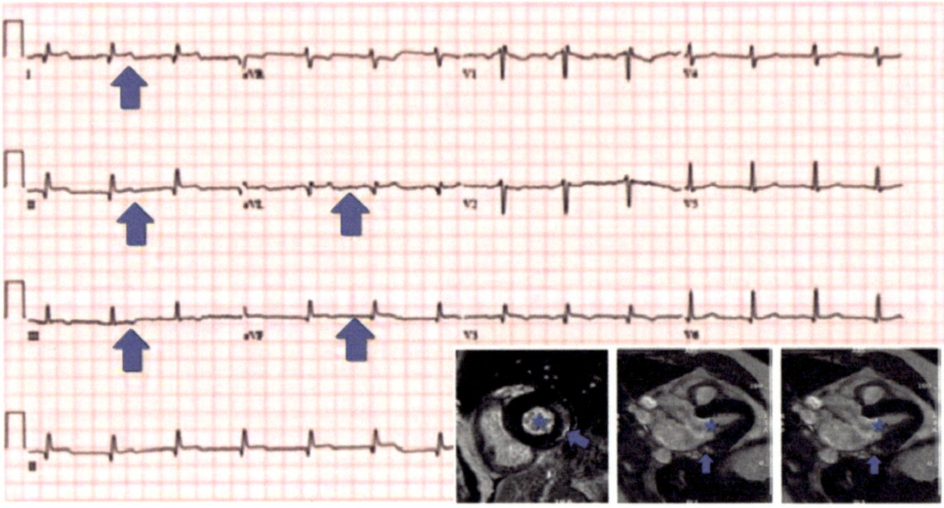

Figure 3.
Findings in a 30-year-old male presenting with substernal chest pain 3 days after he received the second dose of the SARS-CoV-2 mRNA vaccine. ECG: sinus rhythm with nonspecific ST and T wave abnormality lead V3, and infero-lateral ST segment elevations (arrows) with low voltage. CMR scan (bottom right) 2 months post presentation with basal segment, mid to epicardial LGE in the same corresponding infero-lateral and lateral wall territory as seen in ECG findings (blue arrows point to LGE, star denotes the left ventricular cavity). From [51]. Copyright © Sood et al. 2022. Distributed under the terms of the Creative Commons Attribution License.

study including 751 patients with COVID-19, STE were rare findings, while other ECG abnormalities such as the presence of one or more atrial premature contractions, a right bundle branch block or intraventricular block, ischemic T-wave inversion and nonspecific repolarization increased the odds of death [55].

3.3 Imaging

3.3.1 Echo

Echocardiography is often the initial imaging modality utilized in patients presenting with cardiac complaints due to its wide availability and lower costs. It can be performed non-invasively and at a patient's bedside. While findings can be non-specific, it is useful in the diagnosis of heart failure and can determine patterns of dilated, hypertrophic, restrictive, and ischemic cardiomyopathies. It is also effective to easily exclude emergent cardiac conditions such as cardiac tamponade, acute mitral regurgitation, and other states of hemodynamic compromise, all of which may be secondary complications of myocarditis. Myocarditis may cause segmental or global dilatation of the Left Ventricle, focal thickening of the ventricular wall, regional wall motion abnormalities, pericardial effusion, and focal interstitial edema of the myocardium. Right Ventricular dysfunction is associated with increased morbidity and mortality and a higher need for heart transplantation. In a study of 42 patients with biopsy-proven myocarditis, 23% of the patients had evidence of RV dysfunction which was associated with a worse prognosis [56].

Patients with obesity or chronic lung diseases pose a well-known limitation of echocardiography, due to a poor acoustic window which leads to an inadequate assessment of cardiac function and structure [57]. Similar to laboratory markers, the delineation of abnormal echocardiographic findings such as chamber dilatation or reduction in left or right ventricular systolic function as a result of demand related stress from systemic or critical illness (such as from hypoxia, tachycardia, anemia) vs. myocarditis can be a challenge. In general, acute cases of myocarditis have subtle echocardiographic features, including focal wall motion abnormalities and mildly reduced ejection fraction [58].

3.3.2 CMR

Cardiac magnetic resonance (CMR) continues to further advance the diagnostic capabilities possible in heart disease. The lack of ionizing radiation and newer contrast agents that are exclusive of contraindications in those with compromised renal function make it a safe imaging modality to a wider variety of patients. The agent used is often gadolinium, which in a healthy myocardium with intact cellular membranes tends to clear at a higher rate when compared to damaged cardiac tissue. In an acute myocardial infarction, ruptured cellular membranes tend to have delayed clearance of the contrast agent, and in tissues with signs of chronic damage such as myocardial fibrosis the contrast agent becomes confined within the collagen matrix of the scar causing a specific finding on CMR known as late gadolinium enhancement (LGE).

Myocardial fibrosis can be seen in a variety of cardiac diseases oftentimes in characteristic patterns. Subendocardial or transmural fibrosis patterns are often seen after an ischemic event such as a myocardial infarction where damaged tissue becomes replaced with fibrosis. Several diseases have multiple overlapping patterns such as sarcoidosis and myocarditis that can appear with mid-wall or epicardial patterns as a result of reactive interstitial fibrosis. Sparing of the subendocardial border in non-coronary distributions are hallmark features exhibited in non-ischemic scar patterns [59].

The diagnosis of myocarditis using CMR imaging is based on the Lake Louise Criteria. CMR is useful to assess left ventricular volume, size and function, the presence of myocardial inflammation/injury, and the evidence of pericardial effusion. As per the 2009 criteria, in the setting of clinically suspected myocarditis, at least two of the following criteria must be present on CMR to support presence of myocardial inflammation: (1) regional or global myocardial signal intensity increase in T2 weighted images (including evidence of myocardial edema with increased septal thickness), (2) increased global myocardial early gadolinium enhancement ratio between myocardium and skeletal muscle in gadolinium-enhanced T1-weighted images (indicating myocardial hyperemia and capillary leak), and (3) at least one focal lesion of myocardial injury with non-ischemic regional distribution on LGE [60]. It is important to note that with the recent modifications to the Lake Louise Criteria in 2018, the myocardial early global gadolinium enhancement ratio has largely fallen out of favor due to the inconsistent image quality of skeletal muscle to be used as a reference point and two of two criteria were required for a diagnosis of acute myocardial inflammation (**Figure 4**) [62]. Two of two criteria are now required for an MRI diagnosis of acute myocardial inflammation which included (1) myocardial edema (on T2 mapping or T2 weighted images) and (2) non-ischemic myocardial injury (via abnormal T1 mapping, Extracellular volume fraction, or LGE) [63]. Typical findings of myocarditis can be seen in **Figure 5**. The additional findings of left ventricular systolic dysfunction or pericardial effusion, while not diagnostic, can provide additional supportive evidence for myocarditis.

While CMR was a challenge to obtain in early days of the pandemic, follow-up studies on COVID-19 infected and SARS-CoV-2 mRNA vaccine-associated

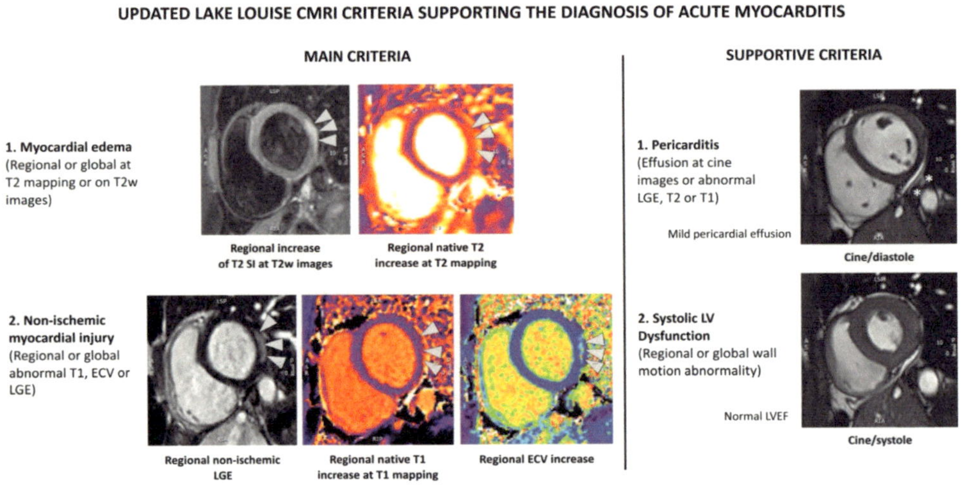

Figure 4.
Case of Acute myocarditis based on 2018 cardiac magnetic resonance imaging Lake Louise criteria. At least one T2 marker of myocardial edema and one T1 marker of myocardial injury are required. On the left: main criteria are fulfilled, as there are both (1) signs of myocardial edema (regional increase of SI on T2w images and regional increase of native T2 at T2 mapping, underpinned by head arrows in the anterolateral wall) and of (2) non-ischemic myocardial injury (regional LGE, increase native T1 at T1 mapping and ECV expansion in the anterolateral wall, underpinned by head arrows, with non-ischemic pattern). On the right: one supportive criterion is present, in fact a small pericardial effusion is evident at cine images, whereas there are neither global hypokinesis nor regional wall motion abnormalities in this case. Abbreviations: T2w, T2 weighted; SI, signal intensity; LGE, late gadolinium enhancement; ECV, extracellular Volume; LVEF, left ventricular ejection fraction. From [61]. Copyright © Elsevier Inc 2020. Reproduced under the terms of the COVID-19 resource center hosted on Elsevier Connect.

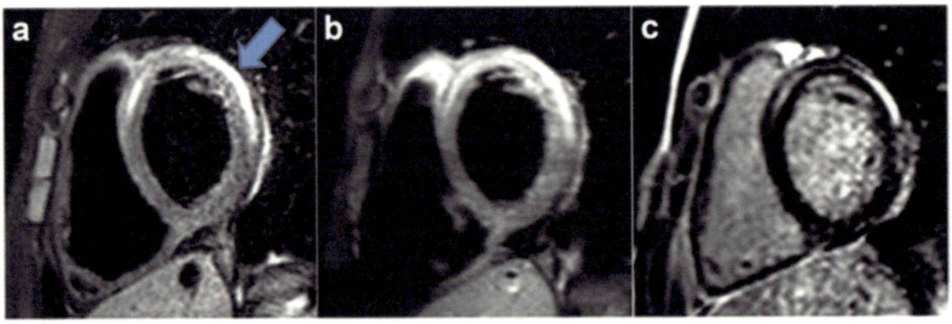

Figure 5.
Typical findings of myocarditis on CMR. 16-year-old patient with midwall and subepicardial distribution of increased signal intensity in the left ventricle (blue arrow) on T2-weighted (a), T1-weighted early gadolinium enhancement (b), and late gadolinium enhancement (c) imaging. From [64]. Published 2015 Nov 17. doi:10.1186/s12968-015-0201-6. Copyright © Banka et al. 2015. Distributed under the terms of the Creative Commons Attribution 4.0 International License.

myocarditis revealed unique characteristics otherwise not seen in other forms of myocarditis (**Figure 6**). A similar pattern of myocardial injury was seen between vaccine-associated myocarditis compared with other causes of viral myocarditis involving the basal infero-lateral wall. However, COVID-19 myocarditis exhibited more widespread fibrosis patterns, such as subepicardial involvement. Those with vaccine-associated myocarditis had less extensive LGE that spared septal involvement [65]. In addition, patients recovering with post COVID-19 syndrome (54%) commonly have cardiac

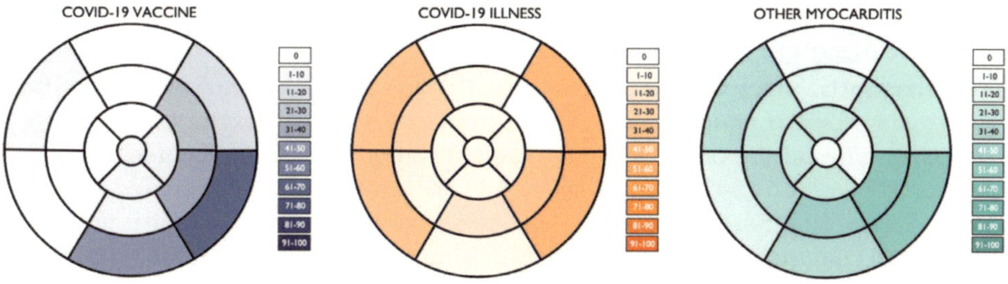

Figure 6.
Segmental distribution of MRI abnormalities. Color-shaded bull's-eye plots represent the percentage of patients in each group with late gadolinium enhancement and/or hyperintensity on T2-weighted images for each myocardial segment according to a standardized 17-segment model. COVID-19 vaccine = patients with vaccine-associated myocarditis, COVID-19 illness = patients with myocarditis who had recovered from COVID-19, other myocarditis = patients with other causes of myocarditis. From [65]. Copyright © 2022 by the Radiological Society of North America, Inc. Reproduced under the terms of the PMC Open Access.

abnormalities: myocardial scar formation (32%), residual pericardial effusion, myocardial edema and interstitial fibrosis likely from persisting inflammation and increased vascular permeability [66].

Five other non-exclusive LGE patterns seen in CMR studies of patients with myocarditis include: (1) subepicardial (common with Parvovirus B19), (2) intramyocardial (common with co-infection of HH6 and PVB19), (3) focal (common mimic of sarcoidosis or neoplasm), (4) transmural (can mimic myocardial infarction), (5) patchy or multifocal (common with co-infection of HH6 and PVB19, or sarcoidosis) [67]. Septal involvement and degree of LGE was found to be associated with worse outcomes and higher rates of major cardiac events, which supports the utility of CMR in prognostication, adding valuable information not only on tissue characterization but risk stratification in patients with suspected myocarditis [68, 69].

CMR is generally appropriate when patients present with (1) new onset or persisting symptoms suggestive of myocarditis (dyspnea, orthopnea, palpitations, exercise intolerance, chest pain), (2) evidence of recent/ongoing myocardial injury (ventricular dysfunction, new or persisting ECG abnormalities, elevated troponin), (3) suspected viral etiology (history of recent systemic viral disease or previous myocarditis). Additional considerations that support a CMR study include the absence of coronary artery disease risk factors, age < 35 years, and symptoms not explained by coronary stenosis on angiogram or a recent negative ischemic stress test [60]. In addition, in patients presenting with new onset heart failure, CMR may be useful in delineating myocarditis from other related or structural abnormalities seen in conditions such as hypertrophic cardiomyopathy, arrhythmogenic cardiomyopathies, left ventricular non-compaction, congenital heart disease with shunt evaluation, or in evaluating other causes of idiopathic dilated cardiomyopathies. This can be of particular importance for the assessment in younger patients with possible vaccine-associated myocarditis who may present with arrhythmias or heart failure and can help guide appropriate management and follow-up, including the return to exercise or competitive sports.

In 2016, the MyoRacer Trial demonstrated the usefulness of mapping techniques in biopsy proven patients with acute symptoms, to confirm or reject myocarditis, superior to the Lake Louise Criteria. In patients with acute symptoms, native (pre-contrast) T1 mapping was a more specific and sensitive test. However, T2 mapping was a superior diagnostic tool in patients with chronic symptoms [70].

In the case of cardiac sarcoidosis and myocarditis, CMR has been shown to improve diagnostic capabilities. In studies, cardiac involvement varies from 0.58 to 7.4%, for clinical diagnosis, which increases from 13 to 45.7% with CMR, and from 24 to 45% on autopsy. Up to 19% of patients had LGE in the absence of cardiac symptoms [71].

Important limitations exist with CMR and specifically LGE. LGE could mimic other nonischemic and ischemic diseases and can be undetectable in healed myocarditis. Falsely larger areas of fibrosis may be present in acute myocarditis where necrosis is in conjunction with edema or absent in mild diffuse disease if separate edema sequences are not performed [72]. Despite the limitations, a subgroup of the ITAMY study investigating the prognostic value of a repeat CMR 6 months after the initial scan demonstrated the greatest survival probabilities in those with complete resolution of edema and LGE, while edema without LGE suggests a residual chance of recovery followed by the worst prognosis in those with residual LGE (especially midwall septal pattern) without edema, likely representing persistent fibrosis [73].

3.4 Biopsy

While the gold standard for diagnosing myocarditis remains histopathological evidence via endomyocardial biopsy (EMB), the invasive nature of the procedure has made the alternative, often a clinical diagnosis (history, examination, labs, ECG)

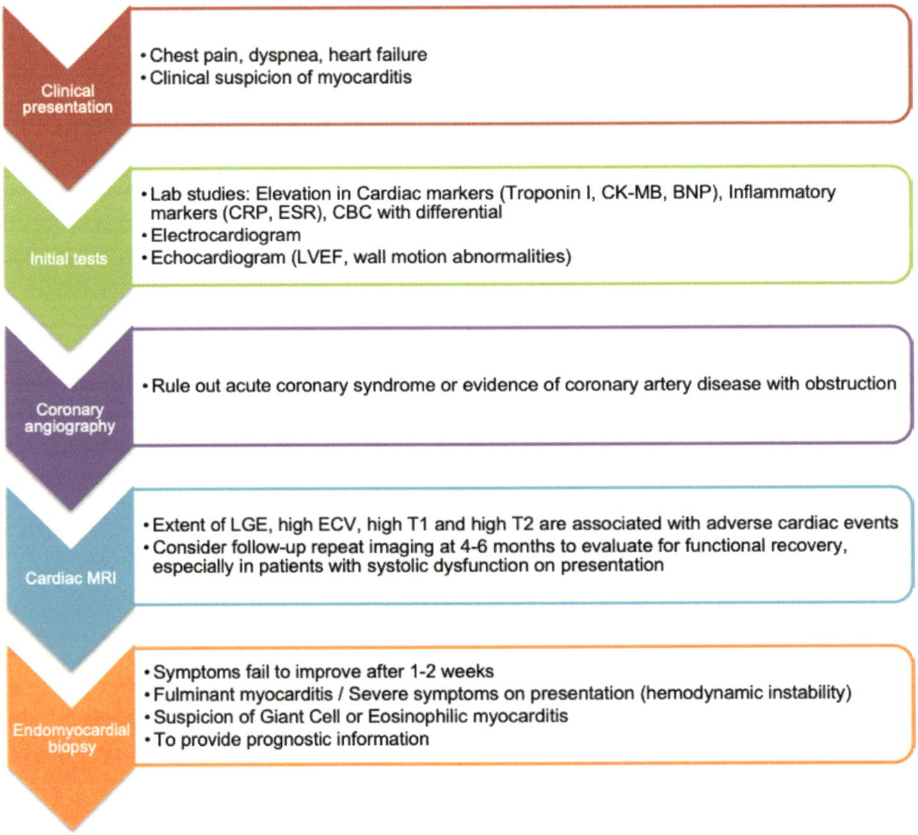

Figure 7.
Clinical and diagnostic approach to diagnosis of myocarditis.

along with echocardiogram and CMR much more common in practice. Biopsy is often reserved in cases of acute myocarditis due to its invasiveness but becomes particularly important in fulminant myocarditis. The initial clinical approach to diagnosis of myocarditis is illustrated in **Figure 7**. An EMB should be performed in the setting of unexplained acute cardiomyopathy (usually a dilated cardiomyopathy) and when other causes of cardiomyopathy have been excluded (ischemic, hypertensive/valvular, metabolic, toxic) in a patient that demonstrates symptoms of refractory heart failure not responding to guideline directed medical therapy, high grade heart block, symptomatic VT or requiring inotropic or mechanical circulatory support [74]. When there is adequate suspicion for giant cell myocarditis, a rare but important cause of cardiomyopathy, death, and transplant, EMB has shown an 82–85% sensitivity on diagnosis [75]. If diagnosed early, it can respond to calcineurin based treatment (cyclosporine) with positive outcomes on treatment course. In contrast, low-risk patients with more benign clinical presentations (hemodynamic stability, mild to normal LVEF >50%, without ventricular arrhythmias or heart block), CMR is preferred over EMB [49].

EMB has the potential for guiding therapy in patients with myocarditis or inflammatory related cardiomyopathies. These patients can be classified into four groups based on biopsy results (**Figure 8**): inflammation-negative, virus-negative; inflammation-positive, virus-negative; inflammation-negative, virus-positive; and inflammation-positive, virus-positive. In addition to guideline directed medical therapy for heart failure, immunosuppressive therapy should be a mainstay for virus-negative inflammatory cardiomyopathy [23]. It should be noted the potential relationship between an idiopathic dilated cardiomyopathy and various stages of myocarditis, thus, it is prudent to delineate the presence of residual inflammation or virus in such patients with a thorough investigation albeit myocardial biopsy and/or advanced cardiac imaging, if clinically indicated. In addition, further research is

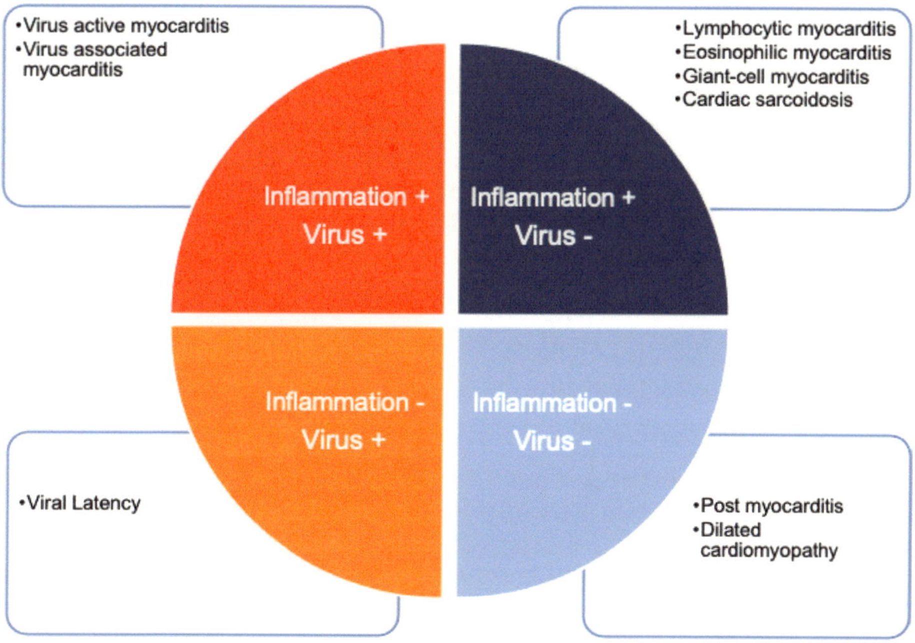

Figure 8.
Categories of myocarditis based on endomyocardial biopsy results. Adapted from [23].

needed regarding the potential role that autoantibody targeting may have in autoimmune, or virus associated inflammatory heart disease.

4. Management/prognosis

In line with the broad spectrum of etiologies, management of myocarditis includes conventional treatment for arrhythmias and heart failure along current guidelines [49, 76]. Tachy or bradyarrhythmia is common in the acute phase of myocarditis or can be asymptomatic. Antiarrhythmic therapy is generally reserved for symptomatic ventricular tachycardia or supraventricular tachycardias that can exacerbate underlying heart failure. Cardioversion can be considered for sustained ventricular arrhythmias. Implantable cardioverter (ICD) is indicated per guideline directed therapy for life threatening arrhythmias or persistent myocardial dysfunction.

Pharmacological treatment is the most common, first line approach including beta blockers for less than class IV heart failure, or the use of amiodarone, dofetilide in refractory cases. Patients that present with hemodynamic stability with sequelae of either acute or chronic heart failure should receive diuretics, angiotensin-converting–enzyme inhibitors, or angiotensin-receptor blockers and beta-adrenergic blockers if tolerable. Aldosterone antagonists may be added for more advanced heart failure with symptoms that persist or LVEF <35%.

The presentation of hemodynamically unstable heart failure may require mechanical circulatory support. In patients presenting with cardiogenic shock where there is severe ventricular systolic dysfunction refractory to medical therapy, ventricular assist devices or extracorporeal membrane oxygenation (ECMO) may be required to prevent multi-organ dysfunction and provide a bridge to recovery by allowing for myocardial recovery or transplant [77].

Patients with myocarditis are encouraged to avoid nonsteroidal anti-inflammatory drugs, alcohol consumption or other toxin mediated substances that have been shown to increase severity of myocarditis. Abstinence from heavy aerobic physical activity has been shown to reduce myocardial demand and reduce the potential for accelerating viral replication. Avoiding physical activity for a period of 3–6 months following the acute phase of myocarditis is recommended with reassessment every 6 months, including the use of repeat biopsy or advanced imaging such as CMR [49, 78].

Current ACC/AHA/ESC guidelines recommend consideration of immunosuppression for patients with active myocarditis and negative viral genome on EMB. A viral genome analysis is generally recommended on EMB samples to determine the safe use of immunosuppressants. Immunosuppressant regimen combinations that include glucocorticoids, azathioprine, cyclosporine is the basis for therapy for giant-cell myocarditis, cardiac sarcoidosis and eosinophilic myocarditis (once drugs or parasites have been ruled out). Patients with a positive viral biopsy for PVB19, HHV-6, CMV, Epstein-Barr, should have initial treatment with antiviral therapy during the acute phase then maintenance with immunosuppression. Ongoing, future, studies for alternative regimens include: the Myocarditis Therapy with Steroids [MYTHS] trial, Anakinra versus Placebo for the Treatment of Acute Myocarditis [ARAMIS], Abatacept for the Treatment of Immune-Checkpoint Inhibitors Induced Myocarditis [ACHLYS].

5. Conclusion

Myocarditis is a heterogeneous disease ranging from mild, self-limiting to fulminant, including the manifestations of heart failure, cardiogenic shock and/or death. While myocarditis has numerous etiologies, viral myocarditis is the most common. Despite an array of clinical, laboratory biomarkers, imaging and biopsy, there is not one sole diagnostic method for its diagnosis. Laboratory markers may provide clues to its diagnosis and their use for continued surveillance may prove useful to monitor disease severity and response to treatment. Echocardiography is a valuable initial modality for the assessment of left or right ventricular dysfunction and to assess hemodynamic instability or secondary complications of myocarditis. Despite the gold standard method of biopsy, it poses several limitations in invasiveness, the diagnostic accuracy based on the location or degree of cardiac involvement, pathological interpretation and resource limitations, and hence, is reserved in refractory cases or those with hemodynamic instability. CMR has superior utility in evaluating myocarditis non-invasively, not only at its diagnostic stage but also in various sub-clinical or convalescent stages of myocarditis and to ensure adequate resolution and follow-up in such patients. Findings in CMR may also overlap with other dilated or idiopathic cardiomyopathies and may be of particular use in conjunction or independent of biopsy. In the new post COVID-19 era, the utility of CMR provides an excellent modality to delineate various cardiomyopathies where an infectious or inflammatory mediated process is in the differential. Clinicians should ensure a comprehensive work-up and thorough surveillance while caring for such patients.

Acknowledgments and author information

The authors would like to acknowledge the Department of Medicine and Radiology at Mount Sinai South Nassau, Oceanside, NY USA.

Michael R. Sood, MD, MS, FACC, FSCMR is the Director of Cardiovascular Magnetic Resonance at Mount Sinai South Nassau.

Conflict of interest

The authors declare no conflicts of interest.

Author details

Daniel Zinkovsky[1,2]* and Michael R. Sood[1,2,3]

1 Icahn School of Medicine at Mount Sinai, New York, NY, USA

2 Mount Sinai South Nassau, Oceanside, NY, USA

3 Mount Sinai Heart – Mount Sinai South Nassau, Oceanside, NY, USA

*Address all correspondence to: Daniel.Zinkovsky@gmail.com

IntechOpen

© 2023 The Author(s). Licensee IntechOpen. This chapter is distributed under the terms of the Creative Commons Attribution License (http://creativecommons.org/licenses/by/3.0), which permits unrestricted use, distribution, and reproduction in any medium, provided the original work is properly cited.

References

[1] WHO Coronavirus (COVID-19) Dashboard. World Health Organization [Internet]. 2022. Available from: https://covid19.who.int. [Accessed: October 31, 2022]

[2] COVID-19 Death Data and Resources. National Vital Statistics System (cdc.gov) [Internet]. 2022. Available from: https://www.cdc.gov/nchs/nvss/covid-19.htm. [Accessed: October 31, 2022]

[3] Aretz HT. Myocarditis: The Dallas criteria. Human Pathology. Jun 1987;**18**(6):619-624. DOI: 10.1016/s0046-8177(87)80363-5

[4] Baughman KL. Diagnosis of myocarditis: Death of Dallas criteria. Circulation. 2006;**113**(4):593-595. DOI: 10.1161/CIRCULATIONAHA.105.589663

[5] Pauschinger M, Phan MD, Doerner A, et al. Enteroviral RNA replication in the myocardium of patients with left ventricular dysfunction and clinically suspected myocarditis. Circulation. 2010;**122**(2):e388. Phan, Mau-Don [added]]. Circulation 1999;99(7):889-895. doi:10.1161/01.cir.99.7.889

[6] Why HJ, Meany BT, Richardson PJ, et al. Clinical and prognostic significance of detection of enteroviral RNA in the myocardium of patients with myocarditis or dilated cardiomyopathy. Circulation. 1994;**89**(6):2582-2589. DOI: 10.1161/01.cir.89.6.2582

[7] Lewis AJM, Burrage MK, Ferreira VM. Cardiovascular magnetic resonance imaging for inflammatory heart diseases. Cardiovascular Diagnostic Therapy. 2020;**10**(3):598-609. DOI: 10.21037/cdt.2019.12.09

[8] Wang X, Bu X, Wei L, et al. Global, regional, and national burden of myocarditis from 1990 to 2017: A Systematic Analysis Based on the Global Burden of Disease Study 2017. Frontiers in Cardiovascular Medicine. 2021;**8**:692990. DOI: 10.3389/fcvm.2021.692990

[9] Cooper LT Jr. Myocarditis. The New England Journal of Medicine. 2009;**360**(15):1526-1538. DOI: 10.1056/NEJMra0800028

[10] Leone O, Pieroni M, Rapezzi C, Olivotto I. The spectrum of myocarditis: From pathology to the clinics. Virchows Archiv. 2019;**475**(3):279-301. DOI: 10.1007/s00428-019-02615-8

[11] Nguyen LS, Cooper LT, Kerneis M, et al. Systematic analysis of drug-associated myocarditis reported in the World Health Organization pharmacovigilance database. Nature Communication. 2022;**13**(1):25. DOI: 10.1038/s41467-021-27631-8

[12] Bellissima BL, Tingle MD, Cicović A, Alawami M, Kenedi C. A systematic review of clozapine-induced myocarditis [published correction appears in Int J Cardiol. 2018 Apr 11]. International Journal of Cardiology. 2018;**259**:122-129. DOI: 10.1016/j.ijcard.2017.12.102

[13] Moslehi J, Lichtman AH, Sharpe AH, Galluzzi L, Kitsis RN. Immune checkpoint inhibitor-associated myocarditis: Manifestations and mechanisms. The Journal of Clinical Investigation. 2021;**131**(5):e145186. DOI: 10.1172/JCI145186

[14] Escudier M, Cautela J, Malissen N, et al. Clinical features, management, and outcomes of immune checkpoint inhibitor-related cardiotoxicity. Circulation.

2017;**136**(21):2085-2087. DOI: 10.1161/CIRCULATIONAHA.117.030571

[15] Ansari A, Maron BJ, Berntson DG. Drug-induced toxic myocarditis. Texas Heart Institute Journal. 2003;**30**(1):76-79

[16] Ferrero P, Piazza I, Lorini LF, Senni M. Epidemiologic and clinical profiles of bacterial myocarditis. Report of two cases and data from a pooled analysis. Indian Heart Journal. 2020;**72**(2):82-92. DOI: 10.1016/j.ihj.2020.04.005

[17] Haddad F, Berry G, Doyle RL, Martineau P, Leung TK, Racine N. Active bacterial myocarditis: A case report and review of the literature. The Journal of Heart and Lung Transplantation. 2007;**26**(7):745-749. DOI: 10.1016/j.healun.2007.04.010

[18] Olejniczak M, Schwartz M, Webber E, Shaffer A, Perry TE. Viral myocarditis-incidence, diagnosis and management. Journal of Cardiothoracic and Vascular Anesthesia. 2020;**34**(6):1591-1601. DOI: 10.1053/j.jvca.2019.12.052

[19] Woudstra L, Juffermans LJM, van Rossum AC, Niessen HWM, Krijnen PAJ. Infectious myocarditis: The role of the cardiac vasculature. Heart Failure Reviews. 2018;**23**(4):583-595. DOI: 10.1007/s10741-018-9688-x

[20] Kallewaard NL, Zhang L, Chen JW, Guttenberg M, Sanchez MD, Bergelson JM. Tissue-specific deletion of the coxsackievirus and adenovirus receptor protects mice from virus-induced pancreatitis and myocarditis. Cell Host & Microbe. 2009;**6**(1):91-98. DOI: 10.1016/j.chom.2009.05.018

[21] Hang W, Chen C, Seubert JM, Wang DW. Fulminant myocarditis: a comprehensive review from etiology to treatments and outcomes. Signalling in Transduction Target Therapy. 2020;**5**(1):287. DOI: 10.1038/s41392-020-00360-y

[22] Lawson CM. Evidence for mimicry by viral antigens in animal models of autoimmune disease including myocarditis. Cellular and Molecular Life Sciences. 2000;**57**(4):552-560. DOI: 10.1007/PL00000717

[23] Tschöpe C, Ammirati E, Bozkurt B, et al. Myocarditis and inflammatory cardiomyopathy: Current evidence and future directions. Nature Reviews. Cardiology. 2021;**18**(3):169-193. DOI: 10.1038/s41569-020-00435-x

[24] Kassim T, Mahfood Haddad T, Rakhra A, et al. A case of amitriptyline-induced myocarditis. Cureus. 2018;**10**(6):e2840. Published 2018 Jun 19. DOI: 10.7759/cureus.2840

[25] Arana GW, Dupont RM, Clawson LD. Is there clinical evidence that lithium toxicity can induce myocarditis? Journal of Clinical Psychopharmacology. 1984;**4**(6):364-365

[26] Maraj S, Figueredo VM, Lynn MD. Cocaine and the heart. Clinical Cardiology. 2010;**33**(5):264-269. DOI: 10.1002/clc.20746

[27] Wilke A, Kaiser A, Ferency I, Maisch B. Alcohol and myocarditis. Herz. 1996;**21**(4):248-257

[28] Raje VP, Lewis NP, Katlaps GJ, Quader MA, Shah KB, Mankad AK. Dobutamine induced eosinophilic myocarditis and right heart failure requiring emergent biventricular assist device implantation. ASAIO Journal. 2015;**61**(2):213-215. DOI: 10.1097/MAT.0000000000000175

[29] Szakacs JE, Cannon A. L-norepinephrine myocarditis. American Journal of Clinical Pathology. 1958;**30**(5):425-434. DOI: 10.1093/ajcp/30.5.425

[30] More LA, Lane S, Asnani A. 5-FU cardiotoxicity: Vasospasm, myocarditis, and sudden death. Current Cardiology Reports. 2021;**23**(3):17. Published 2021 Feb 3. DOI: 10.1007/s11886-021-01441-2

[31] Pallazola VA, Murray JC, Al Harthy M, Zimmerman SL, Webster J, Gondek LP. Anthracycline-induced acute myocarditis and ventricular fibrillation arrest. American Journal of Hematology. 2018;**93**(3):469-470. DOI: 10.1002/ajh.24989

[32] Birchall IW, Lalani Z, Venner P, Hugh J. Fatal haemorrhagic myocarditis secondary to cyclophosphamide therapy. The British Journal of Radiology. 2000;**73**(874):1112-1114. DOI: 10.1259/bjr.73.874.11271907

[33] Wang D, Hu B, Hu C, et al. Clinical Characteristics of 138 Hospitalized Patients With 2019 Novel Coronavirus–Infected Pneumonia in Wuhan, China. JAMA. 2020;**323**(11):1061-1069. DOI: 10.1001/jama.2020.1585

[34] Guo T, Fan Y, Chen M, et al. Cardiovascular implications of fatal outcomes of patients with coronavirus disease 2019 (COVID-19). JAMA Cardiology. 2020;**5**(7):811-818. DOI: 10.1001/jamacardio.2020.1017

[35] Ho JS, Tambyah PA, Ho AF, Chan MY, Sia CH. Effect of coronavirus infection on the human heart: A scoping review. European Journal of Preventive Cardiology. 2020;**27**(11):1136-1148. DOI: 10.1177/2047487320925965

[36] Hamming I, Timens W, Bulthuis ML, Lely AT, Navis G, van Goor H. Tissue distribution of ACE2 protein, the functional receptor for SARS coronavirus. A first step in understanding SARS pathogenesis. The Journal of Pathology. 2004;**203**(2):631-637. DOI: 10.1002/path.1570

[37] Ho JS, Sia CH, Chan MY, Lin W, Wong RC. Coronavirus-induced myocarditis: A meta-summary of cases. Heart & Lung. 2020;**49**(6):681-685. DOI: 10.1016/j.hrtlng.2020.08.013

[38] Shi S, Qin M, Shen B, et al. Association of Cardiac Injury with mortality in hospitalized patients with COVID-19 in Wuhan, China. JAMA Cardiology. 2020;**5**(7):802-810. DOI: 10.1001/jamacardio.2020.0950

[39] Lindner D, Fitzek A, Bräuninger H, Aleshcheva G, Edler C, Meissner K, et al. Association of Cardiac Infection with SARS-CoV-2 in confirmed COVID-19 autopsy cases. JAMA Cardiology. 2020;**5**(11):1281-1285. DOI: 10.1001/jamacardio.2020.3551. PMID: 32730555; PMCID: PMC7385672

[40] Stein SR, Ramelli SC, Grazioli A, et al. SARS-CoV-2 infection and persistence in the human body and brain at autopsy. Nature. 2022;**612**(7941):758-763. DOI: 10.1038/s41586-022-05542-y

[41] Witberg G, Barda N, Hoss S, et al. Myocarditis after Covid-19 vaccination in a large health care organization. The New England Journal of Medicine. 2021;**385**(23):2132-2139. DOI: 10.1056/NEJMoa2110737

[42] Ammirati E, Cipriani M, Moro C, et al. Clinical presentation and outcome in a contemporary cohort of patients with acute myocarditis: Multicenter Lombardy registry. Circulation. 2018;**138**:1088-1099

[43] Aquaro GD, Perfetti M, Camastra G, et al. Cardiac MR with late gadolinium

enhancement in acute myocarditis with preserved systolic function: ITAMY study. Journal of the American College of Cardiology. 2017;**70**(16):1977-1987. DOI: 10.1016/j.jacc.2017.08.044

[44] Vidusa L, Kalejs O, Maca-Kaleja A, Strumfa I. Role of endomyocardial biopsy in diagnostics of myocarditis. Diagnostics (Basel). 2022;**12**(9):2104. DOI: 10.3390/diagnostics12092104

[45] Smith SC, Ladenson JH, Mason JW, Jaffe AS. Elevations of cardiac troponin I associated with myocarditis. Experimental and clinical correlates. Circulation. 1997;**95**(1):163-168

[46] de Lemos JA, Morrow DA. Brain natriuretic peptide measurement in acute coronary syndromes: Ready for clinical application? Circulation. 2002;**106**(23):2868-2870. DOI: 10.1161/01.cir.0000042763.07757.c0

[47] Zhao Y, Lyu N, Zhang W, Tan H, Jin Q, Dang A. Prognosis implication of N-terminal pro-B-type natriuretic peptide in adult patients with acute myocarditis. Frontier in Cardiovascular Medicine. 2022;**9**:839763. Published 2022 Mar 30. DOI: 10.3389/fcvm.2022.839763

[48] Gao L, Jiang D, Wen XS, et al. Prognostic value of NT-proBNP in patients with severe COVID-19. Respiratory Research. 2020;**21**(1):83. Published 2020 Apr 15. DOI: 10.1186/s12931-020-01352-w

[49] Ammirati E, Frigerio M, Adler ED, et al. Management of Acute Myocarditis and Chronic Inflammatory Cardiomyopathy: An expert consensus document. Circulation. Heart Failure. 2020;**13**(11):e007405. DOI: 10.1161/CIRCHEARTFAILURE.120.007405

[50] Patel YR, Louis DW, Atalay M, Agarwal S, Shah NR. Cardiovascular magnetic resonance findings in young adult patients with acute myocarditis following mRNA COVID-19 vaccination: a case series. Journal of Cardiovascular Magnetic Reasoning. 2021;**23**(1):101. DOI: 10.1186/s12968-021-00795-4

[51] Sood MR, Jun-Park W, Imran A. Permanent myocardial fibrosis one-year following the mRNA COVID-19 vaccine: An MRI based case report. Journal of Heart Cardiovascular Medicine. 2022;**5**(1):08-16

[52] Buttà C, Zappia L, Laterra G, Roberto M. Diagnostic and prognostic role of electrocardiogram in acute myocarditis: A comprehensive review. Annals of Noninvasive Electrocardiology. 2020;**25**(3):e12726. DOI: 10.1111/anec.12726

[53] Turagam MK, Musikantow D, Goldman ME, et al. Malignant arrhythmias in patients with COVID-19: Incidence, mechanisms, and outcomes. Circulation. Arrhythmia and Electrophysiology. 2020;**13**(11):e008920. DOI: 10.1161/CIRCEP.120.008920

[54] De Carvalho H, Leonard-Pons L, Segard J, et al. Electrocardiographic abnormalities in COVID-19 patients visiting the emergency department: a multicenter retrospective study. BMC Emergency Medicine. 2021;**21**(1):141. DOI: 10.1186/s12873-021-00539-8

[55] McCullough SA, Goyal P, Krishnan U, Choi JJ, Safford MM, Okin PM. Electrocardiographic findings in coronavirus Disease-19: Insights on mortality and underlying myocardial processes. Journal of Cardiac Failure. 2020;**26**(7):626-632. DOI: 10.1016/j.cardfail.2020.06.005

[56] Pinamonti B, Alberti E, Cigalotto A, et al. Echocardiographic findings in myocarditis. The American Journal

of Cardiology. 1988;**62**(4):285-291. DOI: 10.1016/0002-9149(88)90226-3

[57] Malik SB, Chen N, Parker RA III, Hsu JY. Transthoracic echocardiography: Pitfalls and limitations as delineated at cardiac CT and MR imaging. Radiographics. 2017;**37**:383-406. DOI: 10.1148/rg.2017160105

[58] Bière L, Piriou N, Ernande L, Rouzet F, Lairez O. Imaging of myocarditis and inflammatory cardiomyopathies. Archives of Cardiovascular Diseases. 2019;**112**:630-641. DOI: 10.1016/j.acvd.2019.05.007

[59] Becker MAJ, Cornel JH, van de Ven PM, van Rossum AC, Allaart CP, Germans T. The prognostic value of late gadolinium-enhanced cardiac magnetic resonance imaging in nonischemic dilated cardiomyopathy: A review and Meta-analysis. JACC: Cardiovascular Imaging. 2018;**11**(9):1274-1284. DOI: 10.1016/j.jcmg.2018.03.006

[60] Friedrich MG, Sechtem U, Schulz-Menger J, et al. Cardiovascular magnetic resonance in myocarditis: A JACC white paper. Journal of the American College of Cardiology. 2009;**53**(17):1475-1487. DOI: 10.1016/j.jacc.2009.02.007

[61] Ammirati E, Veronese G, Bottiroli M, et al. Update on acute myocarditis. Trends in Cardiovascular Medicine. 2021;**31**(6):370-379. DOI: 10.1016/j.tcm.2020.05.008

[62] Luetkens JA, Faron A, Isaak A, et al. Comparison of Original and 2018 Lake Louise criteria for diagnosis of acute myocarditis: Results of a validation cohort, Radiology Cardiothoracic Imaging 2019;1(3):e190010. doi:10.1148/ryct.2019190010

[63] Ferreira VM, Schulz-Menger J, Holmvang G, et al. Cardiovascular magnetic resonance in nonischemic myocardial inflammation: Expert recommendations. Journal of the American College of Cardiology. 2018;**72**(24):3158-3176. DOI: 10.1016/j.jacc.2018.09.072

[64] Banka P, Robinson JD, Uppu SC, et al. Cardiovascular magnetic resonance techniques and findings in children with myocarditis: a multicenter retrospective study. Journal of Cardiovascular Magnetic Resoning. 2015;**17**:96

[65] Fronza M, Thavendiranathan P, Chan V, et al. Myocardial injury pattern at MRI in COVID-19 vaccine-associated myocarditis. Radiology. 2022;**304**(3):553-562. DOI: 10.1148/radiol.212559

[66] Friedrich MG, Cooper LT. What we (don't) know about myocardial injury after COVID-19. European Heart Journal. 2021;**42**(19):1879-1882. DOI: 10.1093/eurheartj/ehab145. PMID: 33713116; PMCID: PMC8108615

[67] Mahrholdt H, Wagner A, Deluigi CC, et al. Presentation, patterns of myocardial damage, and clinical course of viral myocarditis. Circulation. 2006;**114**(15):1581-1590. DOI: 10.1161/CIRCULATIONAHA.105.606509

[68] Chopra H, Arangalage D, Bouleti C, et al. Prognostic value of the infarct- and non-infarct like patterns and cardiovascular magnetic resonance parameters on long-term outcome of patients after acute myocarditis. International Journal of Cardiology. 2016;**212**:63-69. DOI: 10.1016/j.ijcard.2016.03.004

[69] Gräni C, Eichhorn C, Bière L, et al. Prognostic Value of Cardiac Magnetic Resonance Tissue Characterization in Risk Stratifying Patients with Suspected Myocarditis. Journal of the American College of Cardiology. 2017;**70**(21):2736. DOI: 10.1016/j.jacc.2017.08.050

[70] Lurz P, Luecke C, Eitel I, et al. Comprehensive cardiac magnetic resonance imaging in patients with suspected myocarditis: The MyoRacer-trial. Journal of the American College of Cardiology. 2016;**67**(15):1800-1811. DOI: 10.1016/j.jacc.2016.02.013

[71] Cheng CY, Baritussio A, Giordani AS, Iliceto S, Marcolongo R, Caforio ALP. Myocarditis in systemic immune-mediated diseases: Prevalence, characteristics and prognosis. A systematic review. Autoimmune Review. 2022;**21**(4):103037. DOI: 10.1016/j.autrev.2022.103037

[72] Luetkens JA, Homsi R, Dabir D, et al. Comprehensive Cardiac Magnetic Resonance for Short-Term Follow-Up in Acute Myocarditis. Journal of the American Heart Association. 2016;**5**(7):e003603. DOI: 10.1161/JAHA.116.003603

[73] Aquaro GD, Ghebru Habtemicael Y, Camastra G, et al. Prognostic value of repeating cardiac magnetic resonance in patients with acute myocarditis. Journal of the American College of Cardiology. 2019;**74**(20):2439-2448. DOI: 10.1016/j.jacc.2019.08.1061

[74] Bozkurt B, Colvin M, Cook J, et al. Current diagnostic and treatment strategies for specific dilated cardiomyopathies: A Scientific Statement from the American Heart Association. Circulation. 2016;**134**(23):e579-e646. DOI: 10.1161/CIR.0000000000000455

[75] Cooper LT Jr. Giant cell myocarditis: Diagnosis and treatment. Herz. 2000;**25**(3):291-298. DOI: 10.1007/s000590050023

[76] Tschöpe C, Cooper LT, Torre-Amione G, Van Linthout S. Management of myocarditis-related cardiomyopathy in adults. Circulation Research. 2019;**124**(11):1568-1583. DOI: 10.1161/CIRCRESAHA.118.313578

[77] Caforio AL, Pankuweit S, Arbustini E, et al. Current state of knowledge on aetiology, diagnosis, management, and therapy of myocarditis: A position statement of the European Society of Cardiology Working Group on Myocardial and Pericardial Diseases. European Heart Journal. 2013;**34**(33):2636-2648d. DOI: 10.1093/eurheartj/eht210

[78] Maron BJ, Udelson JE, Bonow RO, et al. Eligibility and disqualification recommendations for competitive athletes with cardiovascular abnormalities: Task force 3: Hypertrophic cardiomyopathy, Arrhythmogenic right ventricular cardiomyopathy and other cardiomyopathies, and myocarditis: A scientific statement from the American Heart Association and American College of Cardiology. Circulation. 2015;**132**(22):e273-e280. DOI: 10.1161/CIR.0000000000000239

Section 6

General Principles of the Management of Chronic Pericarditis

Chapter 7

Chronic Constrictive Pericarditis

Onur Benli

Abstract

Constrictive pericarditis is the result of a chronic inflammation of the pericardium. Chronic constrictive pericarditis is still a rare disease but is being recognized more frequently. It is characterized by fibrous thickening and calcification of pericardium that impairs diastolic filling, reduced cardiac output, and ultimately leads to diastolic heart failure. Clinically, chronic constrictive pericarditis is characterized by dyspnea during exercise, symptoms of right heart failure. Pericardiectomy with complete decortication is the treatment of choice for constrictive pericarditis.

Keywords: pericardium, constrictive, pericarditis, pericardiectomy, decortication

1. Introduction

Normal pericardium consists of an outer sac or fibrous- parietal- pericardium and an inner double-layered sac called the serous -visseral- pericardium.The layers of serous pericardium include the visseral layer or epicardium,which covers the heart and proximal great vessels. The fibrous parietal pericardium, which contains collagen and elastin fiber and is normally ≤2 mm thick. The visseral pericardium is composed of a single layer of mesothelial cells with accompanying collagen and elastin,which adheres to the epicardium. The visceral and parietal layers are separated by the pericardial cavity, which in healthy people contains up to 50 mL of physiological pericardial serous fluid. The pericardium serves a variety of functions. In addition to its mechanical effects on the heart (limiting distention, promoting chamber – coupling interaction, maintaining cardiac geometry, enabling fictionless movement, hemodynamic effect on the atria and ventricles myocardial and serving as a barrier to infection), the pericardium has immunologic, vasomotor, paracrine, and fibrinolytic activities. However, due to the close proximity to the myocardium, alternations in pericardial elasticity thickness, and volume of pericardial fluid can cause compromise of cardiac filling resulting in pericardial constriction or tamponade.

Constrictive pericarditis occurs with severe fibrotic and cicatricial thickening of the pericardium, loss of elasticity, calcification, and adhesions in the pericardial cavity. Diastolic heart failure occurs as the pericardium, which has lost its elasticity, suppresses cardiac diastole filling. (Hypodiastolia Syndrome).

In conclusion, chronic constrictive pericarditis is one of the causes of diastolic right heart failure. Making that diagnosis may be difficult, as constrictive pericarditis may mimic other disorders. However, constrictive pericarditis is a pericardial disease process characterized by the development of right heart failure secondary to pericardial induced impaired diastolic filling, despite preserved right and left

IntechOpen

ventricular myocardial function. Since it has different pathophysiology, etiology and treatment from other causes of diastolic right heart failure, its definitive diagnosis is mandatory.

2. History

Constructive pericarditis, which has been described as "Pericardial adhesion", "Chronic pericardial adhesion", has also been named as callous, calcified or ossified pericardium, "Concertio cordis cum pericarditis", as a result of knowledge, experience and observations on this subject. This clinical syndrome is also known as "Pick's disease" [1]. In 1669 Lower described the clinical effect of the constrictive pericardium on the diastole of the heart in detail [2]. Based on the autopsy findings of a 30-year-old woman with pericardial adhesion in 1669, Lower stated that the pericardium, which should have been thin/translucent, was thickened, opaque and hardened (callous), which would limit the movements of the heart. J. Mayow, in 1674, described a pericardial adhesion as "as if the heart was surrounded by cartilage and stuck to the front", and reported that this condition prevented blood return to the ventricle [3]. T. Bonet, in 1679, said that pericardial adhesion was the cause of palpitation and used the term (cordis tremor) [4]. R. De Vieussens mentioned the effect of pericardial adhesions on cardiac functions in two cases in 1679 and 1715, and stated that the adhesions were of inflammatory origin, not congenital [5]. A. von Haller described pericardial calcification in 1755 based on autopsy findings [6]. G. B. Morgagni described pericardial adhesions and calcifications in 7 cases in 1761 and gave information about the physiopathology and clinic of constructive pericarditis [7]. In 1823, R. T. H. Laénec detected calcification between the pericardial leaves in the autopsy of a 65-year-old patient with exertional dyspnea but no orthopnea, with cyanotic lips [1]. N. Chevers explained diastolic dysfunction in constructive pericarditis and its clinical picture for the first time in 1842 [8]. Wilks explained constructive pericarditis in detail in 1870 [9]. A. Kusmaul reported in 1874 that venous filling in the inspiratory increased in constrictive pericarditis (Kusmaul's sign) [10]. J. M. Charcat reported constructive pericarditis due to rheumatoid arthritis in 1891 [11]. F. Pick mentioned "pseudo cirrhosis" (Pick's disease) resulting from right heart failure in 1896 [12]. G. Daniel and S. Puder drew attention to the relationship between hemopericardium and constrictive pericarditis in 1932 [13]. T. H. Sellors in 1946 [14] and P. While in 1951 indicated tuberculosis as the primary cause of constructive pericarditis [15]. W.G. Bigelow et al. in 1956 [16], H. B. Schumaker Jr. and Rose [17] in 1960, and Fitzpatrick et al. [18] in 1962 reported that radical pericardiectomy was the only method to prevent recurrence of pericardial constructions. C.A. Bush et al. reported that constrictive pericarditis can disrupt hemodynamics even without adherence to the epicardium [19] E. Weil predicted the excision of the thickened fibrous pericardium in constructive pericarditis in 1895, and E. Delorme also showed on cadavers that pericardial decortication could be applied in 1898 [20, 21]. E. Rehn performed experimental pericardiectomy in 1913, performed pericardiectomy in 4 cases of constrictive pericarditis in humans in 1920, and reported that this was the treatment method of choice [22]. It was predicted by C. S. Beck that this type of intervention could be performed in 1901 [23] and helped in the development of the pericardiectomy technique from 1930 [24]. C. S. Beck reported in 1937 as a result of his experimental studies that the removal of the thickened pericardium provided hemodynamic improvement [25].

3. Epidemiology

The prevalence of constrictive pericarditis is not known for certain, but it is a rare disease. In a prospective study of 500 patients followed for a media of 6 years after an episode of acute pericarditis and the rate of development of chronic constrictive pericarditis is 1.8% [26]. The incidence of constrictive pericarditis in patients with idiopathic or viral pericarditis is lower when compared to other etiologies such as rheumatic disease, connective tissue disease, pericardial injury syndrome,malignancy or bacterial infection. In patients undergoing open heart surgery, the incidence of symptomatic chronic constrictive is similarly low (0.2%–2.4%) [27, 28].

4. Pathology

Histologically, constrictive pericarditis typically demonstrates fluctuating pericardial edema, inflammation and fibrin deposition similar to acute pericarditis, rather than the pericardial fibrosis and calcification more commonly seen in chronic pericardial constriction. This results in pericardial thickening in both situations leading to a loss of elasticity of the the pericardium and ultimately constrictive physiology. Although the constrictive, inelastic pericardium is typically fibrotic, calcific and thick, it is seen that the pericardium is of normal thickness at a rate of 18% in constrictive pericarditis [29].

5. Etiology

All of the causes in the etiology of acute pericarditis can become chronic and lead to constriction (**Table 1**) [30]. However, pericarditis caused by some etiological agents, especially tuberculosis, tends to become more chronic. Tuberculosis from these etiological agents; In regions such as China, Iran, and South Africa, it is the dominant cause of constrictive pericarditis with a rate of 22.2–91% [31–33]. A South African institution reported 121 cases of constrictive pericarditis over 22 years (1990–2012) and of these, tuberculosis was confirmed as the cause in 29.8% of cases and suspected in an additional 61.2% of cases. However, tuberculosis was historically the most common cause for constrictive pericarditis in North America; a report from 1962 cited tuberculosis as the cause of 48% of cases of constrictive pericarditis. And at the present time, in developed countries (North America and Europe), constrictive pericarditis due to tuberculosis is very low (less than 5.6%). In these regions, idiopathic or previous cardiac surgery, radiotherapy to the thorax, human immunodeficiency virüs and AIDS old acute pericarditis are more common in the etiology of constrictive pericarditis [34–38]. It is known that there is a relationship between hemopericardium and constructive pericarditis [39, 40]. Radiation-induced "late pericarditis". Constructive pericarditis requiring pericardiectomy develops in 20% of cases [41, 42]. Constructive pericarditis occurs an average of 23 months after cardiac surgery [39, 40].

Recent studies show that changes in gene expression could be directly associated with inflamation and the subsequent formation of fibrosis [43], the key pathological process underlying the constrictive pericarditis. Furthermore, an array of changes in non-coding RNAs, including micro RNAs (miRNAs), long non-coding RNAs(IncRNAs) and circular RNAs(circRNAs) were belived to play a critical role in the relevant molecular

- Irradiation
- Postcardiotomy
- İnfectious

Viral (Echovirus, Coxsackie virüs, Adenovirus, CMV, Hepatitis B, EMN, HIV/AIDS)
Bacterial (Pneumococcus, Staphylococcus, Streptococcus, Mycoplasma, Lyme disease, Haemophilus influenza, Neisseria menengitides, Others)

Mycobacterial
Mycobacterium tuberculosis
M.avium-intracellulare complex

Fungal
Histoplasmosis
Coccidiodomyocosis

Protozoal

- Neoplastic
- Connective-tissue disorders (Systemic lupus erythematosus, Rheumatoid arthritis, Scleroderma, Dermatomyositis, Sjögren sydrome, Mixed)
- Uremic disease
- Trauma
- Sarcoidosis
- Drugs (Kinidin, Procainaide, Hydralazine, Isoniazid, Streptomycine, Cylosporine, Penisilin, Metyserjid)

Implantable cardioverter-defibrillator patches

- Trauma (blunt, penetrating)

Table 1.
Causes of constrictive pericarditis (AIDS: acquired immunodeficiency syndome; HIV: Human immunodeficency virus).

signaling pathways and biological processes leading to fibrosis.Nevertheless, how these molecular substrates mediate the constrictive pericarditis is still poorly understood. High-throughput sequencing and bioinformatics analysis have been widely exploited to identify specific genes associated with various diseases [44]. These interesting findings promoted researchers to explore if there are abnormally expressed genes and sigaling pathways involved in the inflammation and fibrosis processes of Constrictive pericarditis. Molecular biological experiments are neede to further delineate the roles of these circRNAs identified in Constrictive pericarditis [45].

6. Pathophysiology

In constrictive pericarditis, the pericardium leaves are stuck together and the thickness may be 5–6 mm, sometimes more than 1 cm. Focal or diffuse calcification is seen in 50% of cases. Calcification can sometimes envelop the entire pericardium. The heart in this state is called the "armored heart". In constrictive pericarditis, the basis of the pathophysiological event is the obstruction of the diastolic filling of the right heart and venous return. As a result, cardiac output decreases, venous pressure rises and systemic arterial pressure decreases. The pathological process often extended to the myocardium. In this case, myocardial contractility is impaired (systolic dysfunction). In constrictive pericarditis, in contrast to the symptoms in cardiac tamponade, blood and plasma administration does not increase cardiac output. With decreased cardiac output, liver and kidney perfusion decrease. Salt and water retention increases. Increased blood volume and increased venous pressure do not increase cardiac output. Venous pressure elevation causes congestive symptoms and signs. In constrictive pericarditis, although the left ventricular ejection fraction is normal, stroke volume and cardiac output are decreased. As a result, exercise dyspnea occurred. Because cardiac volume is limited due to constriction, cardiac filling and output vary depending on respiration. The right ventricle will not dilate even though venous return is increased in the inspiration. Rarely, right ventricular volume may be increased by a shift (shift) of the ventricular septum towards the left ventricle. This will reduce left ventricular filling and output.

7. Clinical presentation

The hemodynamic changes and symptoms of constrictive pericarditis are shown in **Table 1**. In chronic constrictive pericarditis, patients may have retrosternal pain and palpitations. In constrictive pericarditis, fatigue and exertional dyspnea develop due to low cardiac output. However, signs of pulmonary congestion (orthopnea, paroxysmal nocturnal dyspnea) are not seen. There may be syncope attacks caused by exertion as a result of the cardiac output not meeting the adequate perfusion. Although exertional dyspnea and peripheral edema are common symptoms in most patients, peripheral edema is scarce [31, 32, 37]. Initially, abdominal discomfort, tenderness, pain, and then ascites occur due to passive hepatic congestion (Pick's disease-Pseudocirrhosis) (**Table 2**).

8. Physical examination

Symptoms vary depending on the stage of the disease.

1. The main finding is jugular venous distension. This finding may not be seen in mild constrictive pericarditis and hypovolemic patients [46].

2. Inflate the patient's face and abdomen.

3. Systemic arterial pressure is within normal limits or low.

4. The pulse pressure range is reduced.

5. Contrary to normal, the elevated venous pressure increases further with inspiration. (Kusmaull sign) [47].

6. Diastolic beat can be noticed with palpation. (Diastolic shock).

7. By listening, the heart is usually quiet and S1 and S2 are soft. A high-frequency early diastolic snap sound may be heard along the left edge of the sternum. (Pericardial knock). This early diastolic additional sound occurs as a result of abrupt cessation of ventricular filling [48, 49]. This is a sign of the sudden decrease in the "y" wave in central venous pressure and the response of ventricular filling.

8. Peripheral pulse may be paradoxical. (Pulsus Paradoxus).

Haemodynamic Effects	**Dynamic Changes in Right and Left Heart Filling with Respiration** **Elevation and Equalization of Cardiac Filling Pressures** **İncreased Venous Pressure** **Decreased Cardiac Output**
Clinical Manifestations	Symptoms: Dyspnea on Exertion Oedema Chest Discomfort Fatique Abdominal Symptoms Cachexia Signs: Juguler Venous Distension Steep, Deep Jugular y-descent Kusmaul Sign Pleural Effusion Pericardial Knock Hepatomegaly Ascites

Table 2.
The principal haemodynamic abnormalities and typical clinical presentations associated with constrictive pericarditis.

Pulsus Paradoxus: Pulsus paradoxus described by Kusmaul in 1872; It is a decrease in systolic arterial pressure by more than 10 mmHg as a result of the pooling of the blood expelled from the right ventricle in the lung bed in the inspiration [10]. In summary; It is the exaggerated form of a normal physiological event [50, 51]. Venous return limitation caused by pericardial restriction causes a decrease in systolic arterial pressure of more than 10 mm Hg in inspiration [51–53]. This event is the dynamic between the pericardium and the heart. Explains the clinical findings that occur because the relationship affects the intracardiac volume/pressure relationship at every stage of the cardiac cycle.

9. Palpation reveals pulsatile liver, ascites, peripheral edema

9.1 Evaluatıon

Constrictive pericarditis is not immediately diagnosed with standard tests. The reasons why diagnosis is difficult is because it shows symptoms similar to heart failure or lung/liver disease. Constrictive pericarditis should be considered in the presence of unexplained heart failure, pleural effusion, jugular venous distension, liver disease, edema. In addition to these findings, if there is a history of cardiac surgery, chest radiotherapy/pericarditis, the diagnosis of constrictive pericarditis is correct. Constrictive pericarditis is most often confused with restrictive cardiomyopathy, which has similar findings.

Diagnostic methods initially include ECG, Chest radiograph, laboratory findings and echocardiogram.

Electrocardiography: The ECG is nonspecific. Low-voltage QRS, nonspecific changes in the ST segment, widening/inversion of the T wave are seen in approximately 25% of patients. The P wave may be narrow and bifid. Atrial fibrillation was detected in approximately 30% of them [32, 37, 38, 54].

9.2 Chest radiography

Findings on chest X-ray are nonspecific, but cardiomegaly due to pleural effusion, pulmonary vascular congestion, or pericardial effusion is seen. Pericardial calcification is seen on chest X-ray in 27% of constrictive pericarditis cases.

9.3 Laboratory assessment

The plasma brain natriuretic peptide (BNP) level can be used for diagnosis. BNP is a determinant of ventricular dysfunction and wall tension. Elevation is typical in many forms of heart failure and cardiomyopathy. In constrictive pericarditis, BNP elevation is less than in cardiomyopathy. Hepatic function tests are abnormal due to congestion.

9.4 Echocardiogram

While echocardiography is performed to rule out heart failure, left ventricular, right ventricular dysfunction, and valve dysfunction, it is very important to distinguish between constrictive pericarditis and restrictive cardiomyopathy, which is most confused (**Table 3**). In echocardiography performed specifically for constructive pericarditis; movement-shift of the ventricular septum towards the left ventricle, as an indicator of increased vena cava inferior pressure; Enlargement of the hepatic veins and inferior vena cava is seen. Pericardial thickening, calcification is seen.

A. *Left shift of the ventricular septum in relation to respiration (shift):* A decrease in left-sided cardiac filling during inspiration causes the ventricular septum to shift to the left. This increases right ventricular filling. In contrast, two-dimensional and M-mode echocardiography shows the septum shifting to the right in the expiration. Sliding movement in the ventricular septum is very important in relation to respiration in constrictive pericarditis, and its sensitivity is 93%.

B. *Change in mitral inflow velocity in relation to respiration:* A decrease in cardiac filling of the left side during inspiration is an indication of a decrease in mitral early inflow velocity [55–57].

C. *Reversal of hepatic vein flow in relation to respiration:* During late diastole in expiration, right-sided cardiac filling decreases as a sign of hepatic vein flow reversal. Reverse hepatic vein diastolic flow during expiration is 88% specific for constrictive pericardium [56].

Computed Tomography (CT): Measurement is made for pericardial thickening and calcification in cardiac CT of the heart (**Figure 1**). Pericardial thickening is detected at a rate of 72% and pericardial calcification at a rate of 35% in CT [29]. In addition, defect in the ventricle contour is detected due to pathology-disease in the pericardium in CT [58].

Clinical signs	Constrictive pericarditis	Restrictive cardiomyopathy
Heart size	Normal	Often enlarged
Jugular venous pressure	M view*	M view
symptom of vomiting	There is	There is
systolic murmur	Rare	There is
S3 Galop**	There is	Except for amyloid
Systemic Disease	Tuberculosis	Amyloid,Sarcoidosis
Thorax radiography		
heart shadow	Normal	Normal/slightly enlarged.
Pericardial calcification	50% have it	Rare
ECG		
P mitral	There is	Rare
Atrial fibrillation	There are 33%	Stylish
message defect	Rare	Stylish
T wave	Inversion frequent	Inversion frequent
Q wave	----------------	Pseudo MI pattern is common
Echocardiography		
pericardium	Thick	---------------
Calcification	Pericardial	myocardial
Septal movement	Normal	weakened
CT/MRI	Thick pericardium	normal pericardium

Table 3.
Clinical and examination findings in the differential diagnosis of constrictive pericarditis and restrictive cardiomyopathy (due to significant x and y descents, **pericardial knock).*

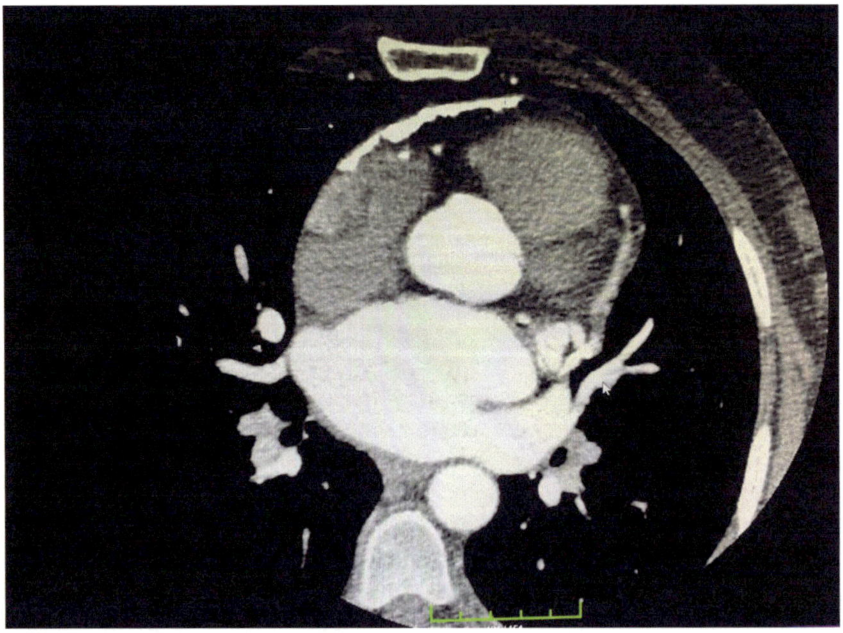

Figure 1.
Computed tomography view of calcific pericardium in constrictive pericarditis.

Cardiac Magnetic Resonance Imaging (CMRI): Provides information on cardiac anatomy including pericardial thickness, calcification and pericardial effusion, such as CMRI, cardiac CT [58, 59].

Delayel gadolinium enhancement (DGE): Granulation tissue and chronic inflammation in the DGE of the pericardium are associated with increased fibroblast proliferation and neovascularization [60]. DGE of the pericardium shows the presence of inflamation, which is a part of the constrictive process, and highlights medical therapy, which is an early -stage option in the treatment [61].

Invasive Haemodynamics evaluation: Hemodynamic catheterization is necessary when non-invasive evaluation methods for CP are inadequate. Especially if the central venous pressure is less than the expected value (less than about 15 mmHg), the sensitivity of the evaluation with catheterization is high [62].

10. Classic findings in catheterization

1. Right and left ventricular diastolic filling pressures close to equivalent, and CVP and intracardiac pressures increased.

2. When the right atrial pressure is observed, deep "y" wave descent and right ventricular pressure "dip and plateau or square root" sign are observed. Both signs occur with decreased pericardial compliance and rapid-early diastolic filling of the right ventricle.

The atrial pressure curve shows high "a" and high "v" waves and prominent "x" and "y" descents ("M" and "W" appearance) (**Figure 2**).

Due to high venous pressure, ventricular filling is rapid in early diastole. The result is a deep fall in early diastole followed by a spike ("tip") and a high diastolic plateau in ventricular pressure curves. This typical finding is called "square root sign" because it resembles the " deep and plateau" and the square root ($\sqrt{\ }$) sign (**Figure 3**).

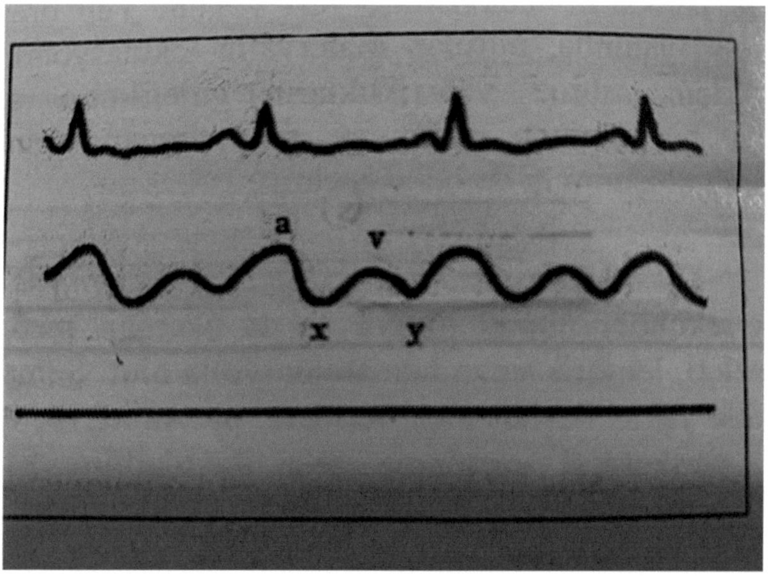

Figure 2.
High "a" and "v" waves, deep and slow "x" and "y" descents (M view) in right atrial pressure curve for constrictive pericarditis.

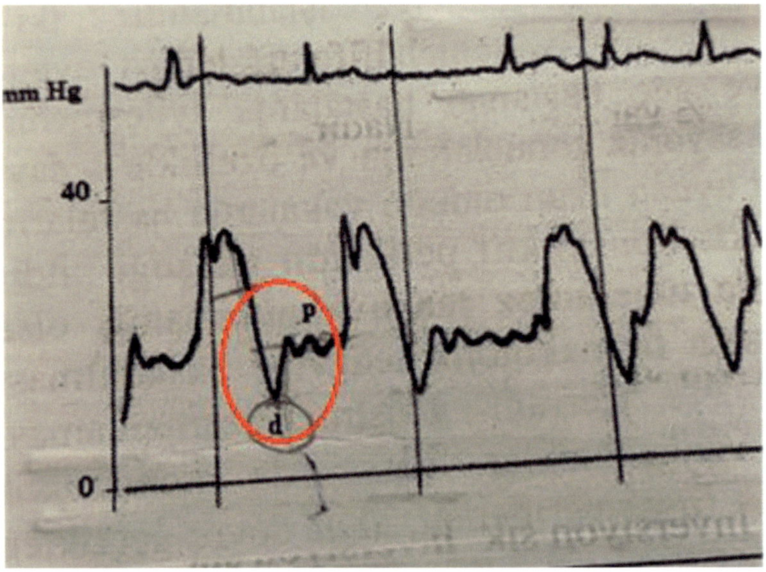

Figure 3.
"Deep" and plateau (square root, indicated by a red elliptical circle) sign in the right ventricular pressure curve for constrictive pericarditis.

3. Right ventricular systolic pressure is less than 50% mmHg.

4. Right ventricular end diastolic pressure is less than 1/3 of right ventricular systolic pressure.

When the gradient between pulmonary capillary wedge pressure and intrathoracic and left ventricular diastolic pressure develops, a difference of ≥5 mmHg between the expiration and inspirum has been reported as 81% specificity and 93% sensitivity for the diagnosis of constrictive pericarditis (**Figure 4**) [63].

10.1 Biopsy and surgical exploration

There may be cases where the diagnosis remains uncertain even after extensive evaluation with hemodynamic catheterization, imaging modalities, and echocardiography. Surgical exploration is sometimes recommended in these cases. Endomyocardial biopsy may be a suitable option before surgical exploration [64] (**Table 4**).

10.2 Treatment

10.2.1 Transient constrictive pericarditis

In some cases of Constrictive Pericarditis, it resolves spontaneously or with anti-inflammatory therapy. In a study conducted at the Mayo Clinic, 17% of Constrictive Pericarditis cases healed spontaneously without the need for surgery [65]. 67% of these cases were temporary Constrictive Pericarditis with effusion. Transient Constrictive Pericarditis most commonly occurs after cardiac surgery. It is also accepted that it may be idiopathic or have infection, trauma or malignancy. Most

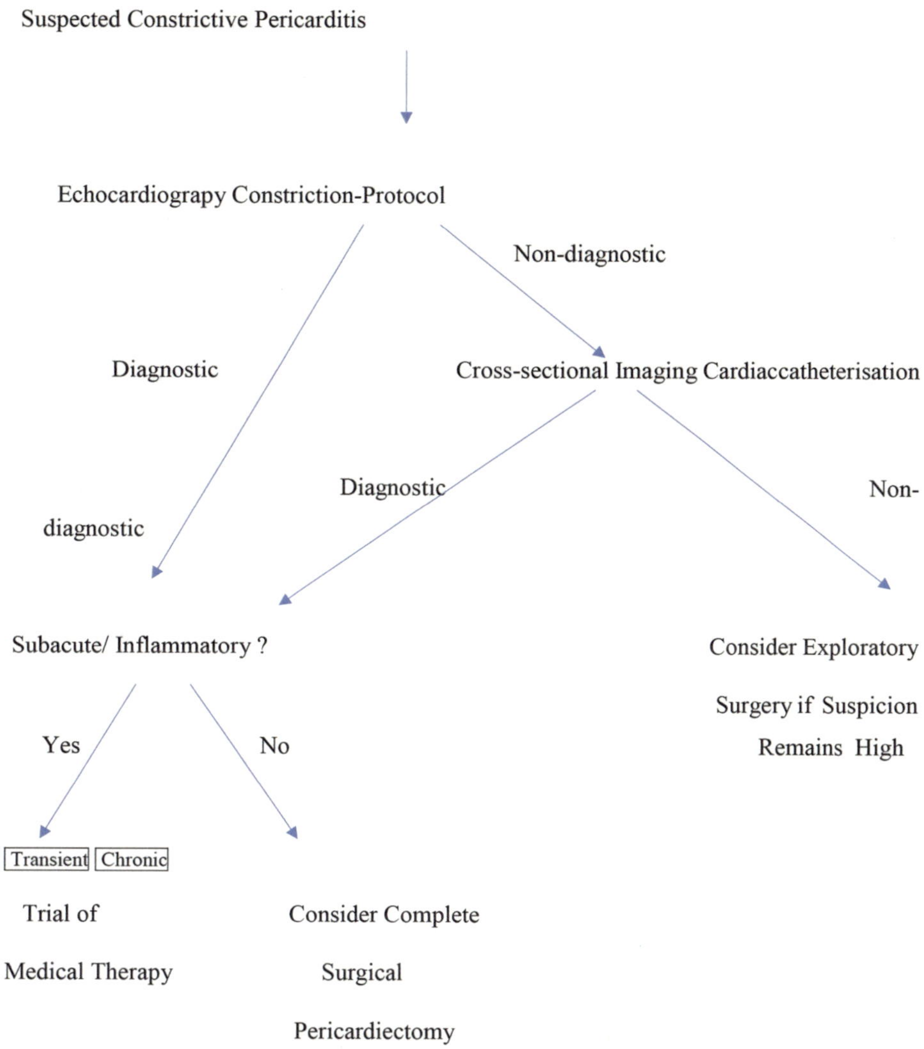

Figure 4.
Simplified diagnostic algorithm for the diagnosis and treatment of symptomatic constrictive pericarditis.

Catheter Finding	Constrictive pericarditis	Restrictive cardiomyopathy
In intracardiac pressures change with breathing	No	There is
Diastolic pressures	Same	LV/RV
left atrial pressure	Equal to RA pressure	It is 10–20 mmHg higher than the RA pressure.
right atrial pressure	> 15 mmHg	< 15 mmHg
"$\sqrt{-}$" ("square root") appearance ("deep and plateau") in the right ventricular pressure curve	There is	Disappears with treatment
RVEDP / LVESP	> 1/3	< 1/3
LVEDP -RVEDP	< 6 mmHg	> 6 mmHg
Pulmonary Hypertension	Light	Intermediate or advanced

Table 4.
Catheterization findings in constrictive pericarditis and restrictive cardiomyopathy.

patients who respond to steroid or non-steroidal anti-inflammatory drug therapy are most likely seen in pericarditis with high serum inflammatory marker levels and high DGE in cardiac MRI [61, 66]. In patients with subacute and distinct pericardial inflamation is reasonable to try 2–3 months of anti-inflammatory therapy [67]. The typical regimen of medical treatment consists of a non-steroidal anti-inflammatory drug with Colchicine or an oral steroid. However, more work needs to be done.

2) Chronic Constrictive Pericarditis: In most of the cases, constrictive pericarditis is chronic and progressive. Diuretic therapy is strictly palliative. The defined and accepted treatment is surgical total pericardiectomy (Pericardial decortication) [67]. Pericardiectomy is an elective surgery. Left anterior thoracotomy is performed by bilateral thoracotomy or median sternotomy. Decortication should be performed on the left and right ventricles, covering the anterolateral and diaphragmatic surfaces, from the phrenic nerve to the other phrenic nerve (if necessary, extending to the posterior of the left phrenic nerve). In this procedure, as much pericardium as possible should be removed (removal) to cover the diaphragmatic and posterolateral pericardium [68]. Pericardial stripping is started from the anterior aspect of the left ventricle and is performed towards the apex. The pericardium over the right ventricle and right atrium is then resected. If the pericardium on the right atrium and right ventricle is liberated first, pulmonary edema will develop as right ventricular output increases and left ventricular pressure continues. Although there are those who suggest that stripping the pericardium on the vena cava and right atrium is unnecessary, the majority recommends that pericardiectomy be performed in these regions as well. Most of the arrhythmias that occur during surgery are due to small infarcts in the coronary vessels. These arrhythmias are controlled with 0.1% lidocaine HCL. Although peeling of the pericardium over the atrium and vena cava is hemodynamically beneficial, the risk is high. To reduce the risk. A cardiopulmonary bypass can be used [69]. Careful care is required in the early postoperative period. Arterial and central venous pressure are monitored. Myocardial insufficiency due to chronic construction does not return to normal immediately after the operation. Low dopamine infusion is started for those with ventricular irritability. Existing hepatomegaly, ascites, edema continue for a few more months. Appropriate diuretics and protein loss are replaced.

11. Prognosis after pericardiectomy

Depending on the prognosis etiology, it is seen that the patient's condition worsens after pericardiectomy in advanced stages of NYHA functional classification, elderly patient, impaired renal function, pulmonary hypertension, decreased Ejection fraction, increased Child Pugh liver disease [35, 37, 70]. Care should be taken not to injure the phrenic nerves during the pericardiectomy procedure. The mortality rate after pericardiectomy is 5–15%, and the most common cause is low cardiac output. The main cause of postoperative low cardiac output is myocardial atrophy caused by chronic constriction; myocardial fibrosis found in cases secondary to mediastinal radiation. After incomplete pericardiectomy, recurrent constrictive pericarditis is associated with an increased risk and reduced survival rate [71]. In the publications of several large volume centers, the mortality rate for surgical pericardiectomy has been reported as 6%–7.1% [34–37]. Long-term survival after pericardiectomy varies greatly depending on etiology and patient character, not age and gender [37]. For example; The cure rate of patients with idiopathic constrictive pericarditis is ≥80% in 5–7 years [34–36]. The long-term recovery rate after surgery is >80% in asymptomatic or mildly symptomatic patients [37]. On the other hand, it has been reported that the outcome after pericardiectomy is very poor in patients with constrictive pericarditis due to chest radiotherapy. The recovery rate in these is 0% - 30% for 5–10 years [34–37].

12. Conclusion

Constrictive Pericarditis; It is a disorder of cardiac filling caused by a diseased, inelastic pericardium that restricts cardiac chamber expansion. Key pathophysiologic feature include dissociation of intrathoracic and intracardiac pressures and and enhanced ventricular interaction. It is a form of diastolic heart failure with different pathophysiology and treatment. It often requires special study as it resembles other forms of heart failure. It should be considered in all patients with unexplained right heart failure symptoms or signs,especially when the left ventricular ejection fraction is preserved.

Diagnosis remains challenging,and the most effective tools are designed to identify the unique pathophysiologic mechanism underlying constrictive pericarditis: dissociation of intrathoracic and intracardiac pressures and enhanced ventricular interaction. Echocardiography is very important in the diagnosis of Constrictive Pericarditis. Methods of cross-sectional imaging are as essential as hemodynamic catheterization in confirming the diagnosis. Cardiac MRI is necessary to provide information about the character of the pericardial tissue, while DGE is necessary to show the presence of significant inflammation in the pericardium and to determine medical therapy(with antiinflamatory).

Complete surgical pericardiectomy has been accepted as the only definitive treatment for patients with chronic constrictive pericarditis.

Author details

Onur Benli
Department of Cardiovascular Surgery, Ministry of Health Adana City Hospital, Adana, Turkey

*Address all correspondence to: dronrubenli@gmail.com

IntechOpen

© 2023 The Author(s). Licensee IntechOpen. This chapter is distributed under the terms of the Creative Commons Attribution License (http://creativecommons.org/licenses/by/3.0), which permits unrestricted use, distribution, and reproduction in any medium, provided the original work is properly cited.

References

[1] Acierno LJ. Pericardial disease. In: The History of Cardiology. Basel Editones Roche; 1994. p. 83

[2] Lower R. Tractus de Corde. London; 1669

[3] Mayow J. Tractus Quinque. Oxford: De Respiratione; 1674

[4] Bonet T. Sepulchretum Sire Anatomier Practica ex Cadaveribus Morbo Denatis. Geneva: Cramer and Perachon; 1679

[5] De Vieussens R. Traité Nauveu de la Structure et des Causes Moument du Coeur. Guilamette: Toulouse; 1715

[6] Von Haller A. Opuscula Pathologica. Lousannae: Bousquet et Soc; 1755. p. 35

[7] Morgagni JB. de Sedibus et Causis Morborum Per Anotomen Indagaitis. Venetiis typ. Renondiniana. 1761

[8] Cherves N. Observitons on the disease of the orifice and valves the aorta. Guy's Hosp Rep. 1842;7:387

[9] Willks S. Adherent pericardium as a cause of cardiac disease. Guy's Hosp Rep. 1870;**16**:196

[10] Kussmaul A. Ueber schwielige Mediastino-perikarditis und den paradoxen Puls. Berl Klin wochenschr. 1873;**10**:433

[11] Charcot JM. Clinical Lecture on Senile and Chronic Disease. 1891. p. 172

[12] Pick F. Uber chronishe ,unter dem Bilde der Lebercirrhose ver laufen Pericarditis (pericarditische Pseudolebercirrhose) nebs Bemerkungen ueber Zuckergussleber (Curshmann). Z Klin Med. 1896;**29**:385

[13] Pudel DG. Pericarditis or pleuritis chollesterina. Cirhows Arch Path Anat. 1932;**28**:853

[14] Sellors TH. Constrictive pericarditis. (Hunterian lecture abridged). The British Journal of Surgery. 1946;**32**:215

[15] White PD. Heart Disease. 4th ed. New York: The Macmillan Co; 1951

[16] Bigelow WG, Dolan FG, Wilson DR, Gunton RW. The surgical treatment of chronic constrictive pericarditis. Canadian Medical Association. 1956;**814**:75

[17] Schumakir HB Jr, Roshe J. Pericardiectomy. The Journal of Cardiovascular Surgery. 1960;**65**:1

[18] Fitzpatrick DP, Wyso EM, BOsher LH, Richardson DW. Restoration of normal intracardiac pressures after extensive pericardiectomy for constrictive pericarditis. Circulation. 1952;**25**:484

[19] Bush CA, Stang JM, Wooley CF. Occult constrictive pericardial disease. Circulation. 1977;**56**:924

[20] Weil E. Traite Clinique des Maladies du Coeur chez les enfants. Paris: O. doin Co; 1895

[21] Delorme E. Sur un traitement chirurgical de la symphyse cardiopericardique. Gaz Hosp. 1898;**71**:1150

[22] Rehn L. Arch Klin Chir. 1913;**102**:1

[23] Beck C, Norburg EP. Some points in the treatment of pericarditis, Journal of the American Medical Association. 1901;**37**:1585

[24] Beck CS, Griswold RA. Pericardiectomy in the treatment of the pick syndrome. Arc Surgery. 1930;**21**:1064

[25] Beck CS. Wound of the heart. The technic of suture. Arc Surgery. 1926;**13**:205

[26] İmazio M, Brucato A, Maestroni S. Risk of constrictive pericarditis after acute pericarditis. Circulation. 2011;**124**:1270-1275

[27] Im E, Shim CY, Hong GR. The incidance and clinical outcome of constrictive physiology after coronary artery bypass graft surgery. Journal of the American College of Cardiology. 2013;**61**:2110-2112

[28] Matsuyama K, Matsumoto M, Sugita T. Clinical characteristics of patients with constrictive pericarditis after coronary bypass surgery. Japanese Circulation Journal. 2001;**65**:480-482

[29] Talreja DR, Edwards WD, Danielson GK. Constrictive pericarditis thickness. Circulation. 2003;**108**:1852-1857

[30] Cameron J, Oesterie SN, Baldwin JC. The etiologic spectrum of constrictive pericarditis. American Heart Journal. 1987;**113**:354

[31] Lin Y, Zhou M, Xiao J. Treating constrictive pericarditis in a Chinese single-center study: A five-year experience. The Annals of Thoracic Surgery. 2012;**94**:1235-1240

[32] Ghavidel AA, Gholampour M, Kyavar M. Constrictive pericarditis treated by surgery. Texas Heart Institute Journal. 2012;**39**:199-205

[33] Mutyaba AK, Balkaran S, Cloete R. Constrictive pericarditis requiring pericardiectomy at Groote Schuur Hospital, Cape Town, South Africa: Causes and perioperative outcomes in the HIV era (1990-2012). The Journal of Thoracic and Cardiovascular Surgery. 2014;**148**:3058-3065

[34] Szabo G, Schmack B, Bulut C, et al. Constrictive pericarditis: Risks, aetiologies and outcomes after total pericardiectomy: 24 years of ezperience. European Journal of Cardio-Thoracic Surgery. 2013;**44**:1023-1028

[35] Bertog SC, Thambidorai SK, Parakh K. Constrictive pericarditis: Etiology and cause-specific survival after pericardiectomy. Journal of the American College of Cardiology. 2004;**43**:1445-1452

[36] George TJ, Arnaoutakis GJ, Beaty CA, et al. Contemporary etiologies, risk factors, and outcomes after pericardiectomy. The Annals of Thoracic Surgery. 2012;**94**:445-451

[37] Ling LH, Oh JK, Schaff HV, et al. Constrictive pericarditis in the modern era: Evolving clinical spectrum and impact on outcome after pericardiectomy. Circulation. 1999;**100**:1380-1386

[38] Avgerinos D, Rabitnokov Y, Worku B, et al. Fifteen-year experience and outcomes of pericardiectomy for constrictive pericarditis. Journal of Cardiac Surgery. 2014;**29**:434-438

[39] Cimino JJ, Kogan AD. Constrictive pericarditis after cardiac surgery. Report of three cases and review of the literatüre. American Heart Journal. 1989;**118**:292

[40] Killian DM, Furiasse JG, Scanlon PJ. Constrictive pericarditis after cardiac surgery. American Heart Journal. 1989;**118**:563

[41] Stewart JR, Fajardo LF. Radiation -induced heart disease. An update. Progress in Cardiovascular Diseases. 1984;**27**:173

[42] Fajardo LF. Radiation -induced coronary artery disease. Chest. 1977;**71**:563

[43] Camporeale A, Marino F, Papageorgiou A, et al. STAT3 activity is necessary and sufficient fort he development of immune-mediated myocarditis in mice and promotes progression to dilated cardiomyopathy. EMBO Molecular Medicine. 2013;**5**:572-590

[44] Liu T, Zhang Q, Zhang J, et al. mi RNA: A database of mi RNA profilling in extracellular vesicles. Nucleic Acids Research. 2019;**47**:D89-D93

[45] Chen Y, Sun F, Zhang Y, et al. Comprehensive molecular characterization of circRNA-associated ceRNA network in constrictive pericarditis. Annals of Translational Medicine. 2020;**8**(8):549-564

[46] Farrar WE Jr. Parzival's pericardial puncture. Annals of International Medicine. 1980;**92**:640

[47] Rajagopalan N, Garcia MJ, Rodriguez L. Comparison of new Doppler echocardiographic methods to differentiate constrictive pericardial heart disease and restrictive cardiomyopathy. The American Journal of Cardiology. 2001;**87**:94

[48] Potain PC. Adhérence général du péricarde. Bull Soc Anat Paris. 1856;**1856**:29

[49] Tyberg II, Goodyear AVN, Langou RA. Genesis of pericardial knock in constrictive pericarditis. The American Journal of Cardiology. 1980;**46**:570

[50] Hitzig WM. On mechanisms of inspiratory filling of the cervical veins and pulsus paradoxus in venous hypertension. J Mt Sinai Hosp. 1942;**8**:625

[51] Mc GM. Pulsus paradoxus. New England Journal of Medicine. 1979;**301**:470

[52] Edmons LH Jr, Hammond GL, Harken AH. Pericardial disease. In: Cohn HL, Edmonds LH, editors. Cardiac Surgery in Adults. New York: MC Grave-Hill; 2003

[53] Savitt MA, Tyson GS, Elbbeery JR. Physiology of cardiac tamponade and paradoxical pulse in conscious dogs. The American Journal of Physiology. 1993;**265**:H1996

[54] Vistarini N, Chan C, Mazine A. Pericardiectomy for constirictive pericarditis: 20 years of experience at the Montreal Heart İnstitute. The Annals of Thoracic Surgery. 2015;**100**:107-113

[55] Hatle LK, Cp A, Popp RL. Differentiation of constirictive pericarditis and restrictive cardiomyopaty by Doppler eachocardiography. Circulation. 1989;**79**:357-370

[56] Welch TD, Ling LH, Espinosa RE. Echocardiographic diagnosis of constirictive pericarditis: Mayo Clinic criteria. Circulation Cardiovascular İmaging. 2014;7:256-234

[57] Oh JK, Hatle LK, Seward JB. Diagnostic role of Doppler echocardiograpyhy in constrictive pericarditis. Journal of the American College of Cardiology. 1994;**23**:154-162

[58] Klein AL, Abbara S, Agler DA. American Society of echocardiography clinical recommendations for multimodality cardivascular imaging of patients with pericardial disease: endorsed by the society for

cardiovascular megnetin resonance and society of cardiyovascular computed tomography. Journal of American Society Echocardiography. 2013;**26**:e15

[59] Thavendiranathan P, Verhaert D, Walls MC. Simultaneous right and left heart real-time, free-breathing CMR flow quantification identifies constirictive physiology. JACC Cardivascular Imaging. 2012;**5**:15-24

[60] Zurick AO, Bolen MA, Kwon DH. Pericardial delayed hyperenhancement with CMR imaging in patients with constrictive pericarditis undergoing surgical pericardiectomy: A case series with histopathological correlation. JACC: Cardiovascular Imaging. 2011;**4**:1180-1191

[61] Feng D, Glockner J, Kim K. Cardiac magnetic resonance imaging pericardial late gadolinium enhancement and elevated inflammatory arkers can predict the reversibility of constrictive pericarditis after antiinflammatory medical therapy: A pilot study. Circulation. 2011;**124**:1830-1837

[62] Bush CA, Stang JM, Wooley CF. Occult constrictive pericardial disease. Diagnosis by rapid volume expansion and correction by pericardiectomy. Circulation. 1977;**56**:924-930

[63] Hurrell DG, Nishimura RA, Higano ST. Value of dynamic respiratory changes in left and right ventricular pressures for the diagnosis of constrictive pericarditis. Circulation. 1996;**93**:2007-2013

[64] Schoenfeld MH, Supple EW, Dec GW. Restrictive cardiomyopathy versus constrictive pericarditis: Role of endomyocardial biopsy in avoiding unnecessary thoracotomy. Circulation. 1987;**75**:1012-1017

[65] Haley JH, Tajik AJ, Danielson GK. Transient constrictive pericarditis: Causes and natural history. Journal of the American College of Cardiology. 2004;**43**:271-275

[66] Cremer PC, Tariq MU, Karwa A. Quantitative assessment of pericardial delayed hyperenhancement predicts clinical improvement in patients with constrictive pericarditis treated with anti-inflammatory therapy. Circulation. Cardiovascular Imaging. 2015;**8**:e003125

[67] Adler Y, Charron P, Imazio M. ESC Guidelines for the diagnosis and management of pericardial diseases: The Task Force for the Diagnosis and Management of Pericardial Diseases of the European Society of Cardiology (ESC) Endorsed by: The European Association for Cardio-Thoracic Surgery (EACTS). European Heart Journal. 2015, 2015;**36**:2921

[68] Syed FF, Schaff HV, Oh JK. Constrictive pericarditis-a curable diastolic herard failure. Nature Reviews. Cardiology. 2014;**11**:530-544

[69] Caccavale RJ, Newman J, Sisler GE, Lewis RH. Pericardial disease. In: Kaiser LR, Daniel TM, editors. Thoracoscopic Surgery. Boston: Little Brown; 1993. p. 177

[70] Komoda T, Frumkin A, Knosalla C. Child-Pugh score predicts survival after radical pericardiectomy for constrictive pericarditis. The Annals of Thoracic Surgery. 2013;**96**:1679-1685

[71] Chowdhury UK, Subramaniam GK, Kumar AS. Pericardiectomy for constrictive pericarditis: A clinical, echocardiographic, and hemodynamic evoluation of two surgical techniques. The Annals of Thoracic Surgery. 2006;**81**:522-529

Section 7

Surgical Approaches to Constrictive Pericarditis and the Post-Operative Challenges

Chapter 8

Constrictive Pericarditis: Surgical Management

Juliana Cobb and Siddharth Pahwa

Abstract

Constrictive pericarditis represents an uncommon sequela of multiple pathologic processes. It involves the pericardium, a tri-layered sac that encases the heart within the mediastinum. Inflammation of the pericardium can lead to formation of fibrous adhesions between the outer wall of this sac and the surface of the heart. Due to the stiff, inflexible structure of the pericardium, its adherence to the heart negatively impacts normal diastolic filling and hemodynamics. Over time, this can lead to reduced cardiac output and severe heart failure. This condition is typically refractory to medical treatment. The definitive treatment of constrictive pericarditis involves surgical decortication and removal of the pericardium to alleviate the constriction and restore normal diastolic filling capacity. This procedure has evolved since its inception and is now the gold standard in curing constrictive pericarditis. However, despite its necessity in the treatment of constrictive pericarditis, this procedure carries considerable risk of intra- and post-operative complications and poor outcomes. The poor prognosis is often related to the patient's pre-surgical status, which must be considered when identifying candidates for surgery. When successful, though, pericardiectomy can produce immediate and progressive improvements in hemodynamic parameters.

Keywords: surgery, constrictive pericarditis, pericardiectomy, surgical treatment of constrictive pericarditis, diagnosis of constrictive pericarditis

1. Introduction

Constrictive pericarditis is an uncommon, diagnostically challenging disease in which the layers of the pericardium become fused and impede normal cardiac function. Historically, the majority of cases were idiopathic. While this is still a leading cause of the disease today, the drastic increase in number of individuals undergoing cardiac surgery, interventional, and electrophysiologic procedures has led to iatrogenic causes becoming a more common source of constriction in the United States and Europe [1, 2]. Elsewhere, tuberculosis infection represents the leading cause of constrictive pericarditis. Studies in India, for example have attributed up to 93% of constrictive pericarditis cases to tuberculosis compared to 4% in one US study [1, 3, 4]. As case numbers continue to rise, the importance of appropriate diagnosis and treatment methodologies will also increase.

IntechOpen

Located within the mediastinum, the pericardium is comprised of 3 layers that encircle the heart. It serves important purposes including protecting the heart from friction-related damage, regulating diastolic filling, and preventing overexpansion. The outermost layer of the pericardium, called the fibrous pericardium, is comprised of dense irregular connective tissue and, due to its lack of elastic properties, helps limit ventricular volume capacity. The fibrous pericardium is anchored superiorly to the great vessels at the base of the heart and is continuous with the tunica adventitia. It attaches to the diaphragm inferiorly. The inner portion of the pericardium is formed by a serous bilayer, collectively referred to as the serous pericardium. The outermost layer of the serous pericardium is called the parietal pericardium and is fused with the fibrous pericardium to form a single outer envelope. The parietal layer reflects around the roots of the great vessels where the fibrous pericardium emerges from the adventitia and covers the outermost surface of the heart as the visceral pericardium. The visceral pericardium is also referred to as the epicardium and provides an external covering for the coronary vessels and myocardial cells. The visceral pericardium also contains mesothelial cells that are responsible for manufacturing and secreting pericardial fluid into the pericardial cavity. This fluid helps lubricate the layers of the pericardium as they come into contact with one another during the cardiac cycle.

Constrictive pericarditis occurs following inflammation or injury to the pericardium. As the pericardium heals, fibrous adhesions can form, anchoring the layers of serous pericardium to one another. This results in anchoring of the fibrous pericardium to the surface of the heart, progressively reducing diastolic filling capacity and leading to symptoms of heart failure. This can be further complicated by formation of calcifications that may extend deep into the myocardium, making cardiac function and treatment more difficult.

Currently, the most effective treatment for constrictive pericarditis is total pericardiectomy [5–9]. This procedure has evolved over the years from the previously favored partial or "phrenic-to-phrenic" procedure which, while less technically challenging, did not resolve all constrictive foci. This resulted in continued constriction of the posterior surfaces of the heart and less-favorable patient outcomes in many cases. With the shift toward complete pericardial resection, survival rates following surgical treatment for constrictive pericarditis have improved. However, the underlying etiology of constriction and patient condition at the time of surgery do play crucial roles in predicting a particular individual's prognosis. While resolution of idiopathic and tuberculosis-related constriction has produced 5-years survival rates around 80%, rates in cases stemming from previous thoracic surgery and prior radiation treatment are much lower [5]. Similarly, patients with advanced disease or poor hemodynamic parameters at the time of treatment experience a perioperative mortality rate of up to 60% [10].

In this chapter, we will review the relevant mediastinal anatomy, discuss the pathophysiology and clinical presentation of constrictive pericarditis, as well as the common diagnostic findings. We will cover, in depth, the surgical treatment of constrictive pericarditis, including the varying approaches and prognostic factors.

2. Mediastinal anatomy

The pericardium forms a 3-layered envelope that surround the heart. It consists of a dense, inelastic outer layer called the fibrous pericardium and a serous bilayer. The bilayer consists of a visceral pericardium that lies adherent to the heart, also known as

DOI: http://dx.doi.org/10.5772/intechopen.109794

the epicardium, as well as a parietal layer that is fused with the fibrous pericardium. The visceral pericardium, comprised of mesothelial cells, secretes pericardial fluid that helps reduce friction as the heart pumps within the envelope.

The pericardium defines the mediastinum within the thoracic cavity, separating the heart and great vessels from the pleural spaces. The pericardium arises from the tunica adventitia of the great vessels superiorly and is anchored to the central tendon of the diaphragm inferiorly. Its lateral borders lie adjacent to the pleura. Anteriorly, the pericardium attaches to the posterior surface of the sternum via weak sterno-pericardial ligaments. The pericardium extends circumferentially to cover the dorsal surface of the heart. Of surgical consideration, the left phrenic nerve lies superficial to the pericardium of the left ventricle and the right phrenic nerve lies to the right of the pericardium.

The reflections of the serous pericardium contribute to the overall anatomy of the mediastinum by creating two sinuses. The oblique sinus spans the distance between the right and left pulmonary veins on the dorsal surface of the heart. This space is encapsulated posteriorly by the serous pericardium and anteriorly by the left atrium. The oblique sinus allows for posterior expansion of the left atrium in to accommodate additional blood volume. The transverse sinus is a result of the visceral serous pericardium reflecting off the posterior pulmonary trunk and aorta to adhere to the atria. This creates an open channel behind the pulmonary trunk and aorta that emerges anterior to the superior vena cava.

The pericardium performs physiologic functions as well. The dense connective tissue that comprises the fibrous pericardium prevents overexpansion of the heart and limits diastolic filling. The fluid produced by the visceral mesothelial cells provides a barrier around the heart to reduce friction during contraction, and the pericardial attachments help to reduce motion of the heart within the thoracic cavity.

The pericardium primarily receives its blood supply from branches of the internal thoracic arteries called the pericardiophrenic arteries. Additional blood supply is delivered from branches of the musculophrenic, bronchial, esophageal, and superior phrenic arteries. The visceral pericardium also receives a portion of its blood supply from the coronary arteries. Venous drainage occurs via the pericardiophrenic veins, which drain into the brachiocephalic trunk and the azygos system. The visceral pericardium drains lymph into the tracheal and bronchial lymphatic chain, while the parietal pericardium empties into mediastinal lymph nodes. Ventral pericardial lymphatics travel over the cranial portion of the phrenic nerves. On the posterior and lateral surfaces, the lymphatics join with lymphatic vessels of the mediastinal pleura.

The parietal pericardium receives somatic sensory innervation from the phrenic nerve arising from C3-C5. The visceral pericardium lacks sensory innervation. Autonomic innervation arises from the sympathetic trunk and vagus nerve.

3. Etiology of constrictive pericarditis

In the western world, acute pericarditis most often lacks a definitive diagnostic origin [5, 11–15]. Of those cases determined to be of viral origin, infection by Epstein Barr Virus (EBV), Cytomegalovirus (CMV), influenza, HIV, Adenoviruses, Echovirus, Parvovirus B19, severe acute respiratory syndrome coronavirus 2 (SARS-CoV-2), and Coxsackieviruses A and B have all been implicated [16–26]. As mentioned previously, tuberculosis is the leading cause of constrictive pericarditis in many areas of the world, though it is not the only bacterial source of this disease [3, 4, 27]. In rare cases, pericarditis may result from bacterial infection by Meningococcus, Pneumococcus, Coxiella burnetii, Staphylococcus, and Streptococcus species [28]. Acute pericarditis may also, in extremely rare cases, be the result of fungal infection by Coccidiodes, Candida, Histoplasma, or Blastomyces or parasites such as Echinococcus and Toxoplasma [29]. The inflammatory reaction induced by these microbial species can lead to formation of fibrous adhesion between the parietal and visceral pericardia, resulting in constriction.

Another leading cause of constrictive pericarditis in western countries is previous cardiac surgery. Rates of constrictive pericarditis have actually increased as cardiac surgery becomes more commonplace and is now seen over a wider variety of age groups compared to previous years [2]. Surgeries in which the pericardium is damaged or manipulated in some way predispose the patient to the development of fibrous adhesions and, later, constriction. Therefore, any patient with a prior history of corrected congenital heart disease, valvular surgeries, coronary artery bypass grafting, or other procedures involving opening of the mediastinum should be evaluated for the development of pericardial thickening or calcification. One twenty-year study found that patients diagnosed with constrictive pericarditis were more likely to have been treated surgically for valvular disease and atrial fibrillation and demonstrated a significantly increased 7-year mortality rate compared to controls [30].

Patients who have undergone mediastinal irradiation for treatment of primary or metastatic cancer are also at increased risk of developing constrictive pericarditis. Some evidence suggests that patients who develop constrictive pericarditis following radiation treatment are also at increased risk of mortality following pericardiectomy compared with patients receiving the same procedure for other causative states [10]. In fact, mediastinal irradiation is considered an independent prognostic factor for mortality following surgical correction of constrictive pericarditis, with 5-year survival at a dismal 11.0% and an increased 10-year mortality rate [13]. One retrospective study reported an overall intraoperative mortality of 10.1% for patients with a history of mediastinal irradiation over a seventeen-year period, though it should be noted that the majority of those patients underwent concomitant procedures that may have attributed to their outcome [31]. While there have been numerous reports indicating poor outcomes for patients undergoing pericardiectomy following mediastinal radiation treatment, it cannot be overlooked that the increased mortality rates among these patients may be related to their original need for radiation therapy, rather than an interaction between pericardiectomy and irradiated tissue.

In developing countries, tuberculosis infection is most often the causative agent of constrictive pericarditis. This is especially pronounced in HIV-positive patients who may lack the robust immune system needed to protect the pericardium from inflammation. Current estimates suggest that tuberculosis is second only to purulent disease as the cause of constrictive pericarditis in areas such as sub-Saharan Africa and Asia [27]. Exact data is difficult to acquire, however, due to the challenges of diagnosing this disease. Definitive diagnosis of tuberculous pericarditis is based on the presence of tubercle bacilli in samples of a patient's pericardial fluid or histologic section of their pericardium. It is possible to identify "probable" cases in patients with known tuberculosis infection and otherwise idiopathic pericarditis [4].

Other, less common, causes of constrictive pericarditis include connective tissue diseases such as rheumatoid arthritis, systemic lupus erythematosus, Behçet's disease, scleroderma, and Sjögren syndrome [7, 32–34]. Amyloidosis and sarcoidosis can result in fibrous adherence between pericardial layers, as can metabolic pathologies such as uremia [35–40]. Inflammation secondary to acute coronary syndromes have also been shown to precipitate constrictive pericarditis, a condition known as Dressler's syndrome [41, 42]. Additionally, purulent pericarditis may lead to constriction in cases of incomplete drainage [41, 43].

Lastly, certain pharmaceuticals have been implicated in the pathogenesis of constrictive pericarditis. Procainamide, hydralazine, and isoniazid have all been reported as causative agents of drug-induced systemic lupus erythematosus (SLE) [33, 44]. SLE, as previously discussed, can lead to pericarditis through the induction of serositis [33, 34]. The resultant inflammation can produce constrictive adhesions in such instances. Cardiotoxic drugs, such as Ipilimumab and Nivolumab, have also been attributed to development of constrictive pericarditis [45–48]. Patients taking these drugs should be monitored for changes in hemodynamic parameters and evidence of constriction.

4. Pathophysiology of constrictive pericarditis

Constrictive pericarditis is the result of a chronic inflammatory process that causes fibrous adhesions and calcifications to form between the epicardium and parietal pericardium. The ongoing inflammation leads to calcium deposition and remodeling, resulting in thickening and scarring of the tissue. This scarring can reach deep into the adjacent myocardium, further reducing cardiac function. This inflammation may be attributed to episode(s) of acute pericarditis, chronic pericarditis, or the other mechanisms described above.

Inflammation of the pericardium can result from a number of processes and occurs in both acute and chronic forms. Acute pericarditis is one of the most common disorders involving the pericardium and occurs in approximately 0.1–0.2% of hospitalized patients and 5% of patients admitted to the emergency department for nonischemic chest pain [49, 50]. Clinical presentation of acute pericarditis includes sharp, pleuritic chest pain that is alleviated with the patient leans forward, thereby decreasing contact of the pericardium with nearby structures. On auscultation, a pericardial friction rub can be heard at the left sternal border. Electrocardiogram changes commonly associated with acute pericarditis include depression of the PR segment and widespread ST elevation early in the disease process. It should be noted, however, that these ECG findings may change over the course of the disease.

Under normal physiologic conditions, the pericardium is not especially compliant but is capable of accommodating small changes in preload experienced by the heart. It can also expand over time in cases of prolonged, slowly accumulating pericardial effusion. However, the pericardium is not typically distensible or capable of elastic recoil. This becomes relevant when discussing the pathologic changes observed in constrictive pericarditis. In the normal cardiac cycle, diastolic volume increases by approximately 70 mL over systolic volume. This expansion in volume causes the lateral walls of the ventricles to expand outward, which is accommodated by the pericardial cavity. This helps to regulate filling volume while also allowing for appropriate preload.

Another part of normal physiology is the interplay between respiration and cardiac filling. This is represented by the relationship between intrathoracic and intracardiac pressures. During inspiration, there is an increase in right-sided venous return, which causes expansion of the right ventricle and pushes the interventricular septum into the left ventricle to accommodate the added volume. This produces a transient reduction in left ventricular size and transmural filling pressure, leading to a drop in left ventricular end diastolic volume. Reduced end diastolic volume results in reduced stroke volume. These changes tend to be minimal and produce only small changes to hemodynamic parameters.

When adhesions form between the layers of the pericardium, the pericardial cavity is lost, and the outer fibrous pericardium must move in synchrony with the expanding ventricles during diastole. As mentioned, though, the fibrous pericardium lacks elasticity. This limits the ability of the ventricle to expand outwardly and accommodate its normal diastolic volume. As the constriction becomes more severe, ventricular filling can become severely impeded and even lead to transient displacement of the interventricular septum into the left ventricle, called septal bounce. Decreasing the preload capacity of the heart leads to reduced cardiac output and venous congestion. Over time, the restricted ventricular filling leads to dissociation of intracardiac and intrathoracic pressures with respiration and equalization of intracardiac diastolic filling pressures, which increase until the patient develops right heart dysfunction [51]. Reductions in caval flow velocity during expiration, decreased mitral flow velocity, reduced heart rate, and increased hepatic venous diastolic flow also result [52]. Reduced end diastolic volume, stroke volume, and cardiac output result. These changes mimic, and can eventually lead to, heart failure.

5. Patient presentation and symptom progression

Patients with constrictive pericarditis often present with symptoms that mimic heart failure with preserved ejection fraction. As adhesions form between the parietal pericardium and epicardium, myocardial function is progressively hindered. This results in reduced cardiac output as well as pulmonary and systemic venous congestion. These abnormal physiologies can lead to symptoms of progressive exertional dyspnea, fatigue, tachypnea, peripheral edema, and gastrointestinal upset [1, 7, 53]. The patient may also experience exertion-independent tachycardia. Some patients may report chest pain or present with atrial arrhythmias, or symptoms of cardiac tamponade [1, 7, 53].

It is important to obtain a thorough patient history in a patient presenting with signs of heart failure. Those who report previous episodes of acute pericarditis, tuberculosis, mediastinal radiation treatment, prior cardiothoracic surgery, or previous chest trauma should produce a high index of suspicion for constrictive pericarditis.

5.1 Physical exam

Constrictive pericarditis can be identified on physical exam of the patient through palpation of the precordium. A 'diastolic apex beat' or diastolic precordial impulse represents a positive finding, as this beat should normally be felt during systole [51]. The abrupt termination of early diastolic filling, which is characteristic in constrictive pericarditis, is responsible for this switch. Note that a positive finding should be confirmed by palpating the impulse at multiple areas along the sternum and epigastric region and comparing the beat against the carotid pulse [51, 54].

While precordial palpation can reveal characteristic signs of constrictive pericarditis, the most common, though nonspecific, finding is elevated jugular venous pressure [51, 54]. Distension can frequently be observed by reclining the patient to an elevation of thirty degrees and having them look to their left. The clinician can then evaluate the jugular vein for distension and abnormal pulsation. It should be noted that elevated jugular venous pressure may not be observed in patients with mild to moderate constriction [54]. However, a high index of suspicion should be aroused in patients presenting with unexplained jugular vein distension and a history of known predisposition to constrictive pericarditis.

Other features that may be observed include pericardial knock or friction rub, Kussmaul sign, or pulsus paradoxus [2]. As mentioned previously, peripheral edema is also a frequent finding in patients with constrictive pericarditis, which may be accompanied by ascities and hepatomegaly [51]. Pleural effusion is also often found during the physical exam [2].

6. Diagnostic criteria and the differential

Early diagnosis of constrictive pericarditis is of vital importance to the success of treatment as well as the long-term prognosis of the patient. Early treatment via pericardiectomy is associated with lower intra- and post-operative risk and reduced incidence of complications [51]. Surgical intervention prior to the onset of NYHA Class III or IV symptoms—that is, heart failure symptoms with minimal exertion or at rest, respectively, is associated with significantly reduced risk of morbidity and mortality in the 30-days following pericardiectomy [7, 51, 55].

6.1 Imaging

The diagnosis of constrictive pericarditis is based on guidelines set by the American College of Cardiology and the European Society of Cardiology, both of which recommend evaluation by 2-D echocardiogram [7, 56]. This test allows for visualization of calcifications or increased thickness of the pericardium—both diagnostic indicators of constrictive pericarditis. Echocardiogram also detects two other characteristic changes associated with constriction: ventricular interdependence and loss of intrathoracic pressure variation with breathing [7, 10, 56–58]. The abnormal rigidity of the pericardium in constrictive pericarditis prevents independent activity of the ventricles, which can be seen as decreased diastolic filling time and septal bounce [7, 10, 56–58]. Additionally, echocardiogram may detect the presence of dilation of the inferior vena cava due to decreased preload [7, 10, 56–58].

M-mode ultrasound may also be used to exclude constrictive pericarditis from a list of differential diagnoses. In constrictive pericarditis, when a patient inhales, M-mode ultrasound should show posterior movement of the interventricular septum during the early diastolic phase [59–61]. Another inspiratory feature indicative of pericardial constriction is the absence of increased systemic venous return, again visible on ultrasound [61, 62]. A third feature that would suggest a patient may be experiencing constrictive pericarditis is the premature opening of the pulmonic valve due to increased ventricular diastolic pressure [61, 62]. Absence of any of these three features should help the clinician to rule out constrictive pericarditis [61].

Doppler echocardiography is also useful in the diagnosis of constrictive pericarditis. Key indicators of this state include abnormal filling of the ventricles in early diastole and changes in flow velocity across the tricuspid valve during the respiratory cycle [63–65]. More specifically, during inspiration the clinician should expect to see an increase in diastolic flow velocity followed by a decrease during expiration [56]. Additionally, the pulmonary veins and mitral valve should experience a drastic reduction in flow velocity during inspiration accompanied by a shift of the interventricular septum toward the left ventricle [56].

Computed tomography (CT) and cardiovascular magnetic resonance (CMR) imaging are commonly used as adjuncts to echocardiography when making a definitive diagnosis of constrictive pericarditis. These imaging modalities are particularly useful, though, in differentiating constrictive pericarditis from restrictive cardiomyopathy, a challenging distinction and common misdiagnosis. Cardiac MRI and CT provide higher resolution and a broader field of view than more traditional imaging modalities [66]. Cardiac MRI, in particular, is able to provide high-resolution and contrast of the heart and related cardiac structures, including the pericardium. Use of cardiac MRI allows for accurate measurement of pericardial thickness, which can be used as diagnostic criteria in constrictive pericarditis. Pericardium that exceeds 4 mm in thickness produces a signal intensity that is equal to that of the myocardium and characteristic calcification of the tissue can be visualized as well [67]. Other abnormalities associated with constrictive pericarditis that may be detected with cardiac MRI include "tubing" of the right ventricle, enlargement of the atria, abnormal motion of the interventricular septum, and enlargement of the inferior vena cava due to decreased preload [67].

Chest radiographs may also be useful in the diagnosis of constrictive pericarditis. Patients who exhibit calcifications on radiograph in the presence of a consistent clinical picture should produce a high index of suspicion. More specifically, lateral and anterior oblique images of patients with constrictive pericarditis may show concentric, linear rings of calcification surrounding the heart [7]. It should be noted that evidence of pericardial calcifications on chest radiograph is not in itself diagnostic of constrictive pericarditis as calcification can occur for a number of reasons, however the pattern in non-constrictive disease is often more diffuse or patchy [7, 68, 69]. Some patients with constrictive pericarditis may not show evidence of calcification at all and therefore radiograph should not be used to eliminate this diagnosis from the differential in the setting of other, more characteristic findings.

6.2 Electrocardiogram

In contrast to acute pericarditis, constrictive pericarditis does not demonstrate pathognomonic changes on electrocardiogram (ECG). A wide variety of ECG changes, ranging from a normal QRS complex to low voltage, and generalized T-wave flattening, or inversion may be exhibited [70]. Other commonly seen ECG changes are those of right ventricular hypertrophy and right axis deviation [70]. Some patients may display non-specific ST-segment changes, but the most common abnormality observed is low voltage but, as stated, this is not diagnostic of constriction. Also, in patients with long-standing or advanced constriction, the chronic elevation of left atrial pressures may manifest as atrial fibrillation [6, 71]. While ECG findings may aid in the diagnosis of constrictive pericarditis, any changes should be evaluated in conjunction with echocardiography and CT or CMR imaging.

6.3 Cardiac catheterization

While more noninvasive diagnostic techniques are generally favored in the diagnosis of constrictive pericarditis, right heart catheterization remains the gold standard and should be performed in patients being considered for surgical treatment. Cardiac catheterization is particularly useful when other imaging modalities produce inconclusive results, or the diagnosis is particularly challenging. Cardiac catheterization allows for monitoring of the hemodynamic changes characteristic of constrictive pericarditis. In particular, the abnormal ventricular filling associated with different phases of the respiratory cycle and eventual equalization and interdependence of right and left diastolic pressures can be measured with cardiac catheterization, then used in the making of a definitive diagnosis [72].

Pressure changes during cardiac catheterization can also be of substantial use in confirming a diagnosis of constrictive pericarditis. Indications include a notable drop in pulmonary capillary wedge pressure compared to left ventricular diastolic pressure during inspiration and sharp decreases in x and y descents of atrial and venous pressure tracings [7, 73]. Diastolic pressure changes in the right and left ventricles may produce a "square root" sign with an absent wave, which reflects the rapid ventricular filling during early diastole, followed by diastatic plateau caused by compression [7]. Findings may also include increased right atrial pressure and increased right ventricular end-diastolic pressure [7].

6.4 Differential diagnoses

Diagnosis of constrictive pericarditis can be particularly challenging as the clinical presentation of this disease closely resembles heart failure with preserved ejection fraction, which can have a number of underlying etiologies. Therefore, it is important for clinicians to maintain a high index of suspicion in patients who report predisposing factors, such as prior cardiothoracic surgery, previous mediastinal radiation or malignancy, thoracic trauma, tuberculosis, or a history of connective tissue disorders (see Section 3). A thorough physical exam and utilization of the imaging modalities described above can help to rule in or rule out a diagnosis of constrictive pericarditis. Still, definitive diagnosis can be difficult.

On the list of differentials in a patient presenting with signs of constrictive pericarditis should be restrictive cardiomyopathy. While constrictive pericarditis results from pericardial thickening and formation of adhesions between pericardial layers that results in reduced ventricular compliance, restrictive cardiomyopathy is due to progressive myocardial stiffness which likewise produces a decrease in ventricular compliance. Restrictive cardiomyopathy is often considered to be the most diagnostically similar to constrictive pericarditis and may therefore be difficult identify. Proper differentiation between these two conditions is crucial, as the treatment methodologies vary drastically. Constrictive pericarditis, in many cases, can undergo definitive treatment with pericardiectomy. Restrictive cardiomyopathy, on the other hand, has no curative therapeutic options and often requires cardiac transplantation.

As mentioned previously, constrictive pericarditis is frequently associated with a history of one or more predisposing factors. Prior treatment for mediastinal malignancy, mediastinal radiation, or with cardiothoracic surgery should increase suspicion of underlying constriction [5, 7, 11, 12, 15, 74]. Likewise, constrictive pericarditis, unlike restrictive cardiomyopathy, is associated with a history of tuberculosis, viral infections, trauma, and connective tissue disease [17, 18, 20, 22–26, 75]. Restrictive cardiomyopathy, in contrast, is often related to sarcoidosis, amyloidosis, or inherited mutations in one of several genes related to the sarcomere subunit [6].

In both constrictive pericarditis and restrictive cardiomyopathy, patients can have increased right and left sided filling pressures and preserved ejection fractions [6, 7]. Both conditions can also present as diastolic heart failure in their later stages [6, 7]. Fortunately, appropriate diagnostic testing and a thorough patient history can help elucidate the underlying cause of a patient's symptoms and ensure proper treatment. Though not an exhaustive list, some useful diagnostic differences between constrictive pericarditis and restrictive cardiomyopathy include:

1. Whereas constrictive pericarditis generally lacks notable ECG changes, restrictive cardiomyopathy can present with changes in depolarization, pathologic Q waves, impaired conduction, repolarization abnormalities, or ventricular hypertrophy [76]. Though it may be possible to observe abnormal repolarization or low voltage in constrictive pericarditis though or nonspecific ST or T wave changes, again, this is not common [60]. Also of note, in their later stages both conditions may predispose a patient to atrial fibrillation [6, 71].

2. The difference in the underlying pathophysiology of both diseases produces varying results in B-type natriuretic peptide (BNP) values and imaging studies. BNP levels tend to be higher in patients experiencing restrictive cardiomyopathy compared to constrictive pericarditis, likely owing to lack of ventricular wall compliance in the former [77–79].

3. Pericardial calcification is sometimes seen in constrictive pericarditis but has not been commonly associated with restrictive cardiomyopathy [7, 68, 69]. Rarely, calcification of the ventricle may be seen in restrictive physiology and may contribute to the pathogenesis of this disease [80].

4. Perhaps of no surprise, pericardial changes are not commonly observed in the setting of restrictive cardiomyopathy [81]. Increased pericardial thickness (>4 mm) may, however, be indicative of constrictive pericarditis when seen on imaging [60]. It should be noted that pericardial thickening is not always observed in patients with constrictive pericarditis and the absence of thickening should not be used to definitively eliminate constriction from the differential [60, 81].

5. As mentioned previously, constrictive pericarditis frequently presents with significant respiration-dependent changes in ventricular filling on Doppler studies [82]. Any such filling changes in restrictive cardiomyopathy are usually minimal [82]. When measuring pulmonary venous flow using transesophageal echocardiography, it has been reported that peak systolic flow variations and flow velocities during the respiratory cycle were also greater in patients with confirmed constrictive pericarditis, comparted with restrictive cardiomyopathy [65].

6. The fibrous myocardium that is characteristic of restrictive cardiomyopathy limits movement of the muscle. This is translated into markedly reduced septal bounce during diastole. As discussed previously, constrictive pericarditis produces notably increased septal bounce as movement of the outer walls of the ventricle become more impeded [7, 10, 56–58].

7. Measures of tissue strain using CMR tend to be significantly higher in patients with restrictive cardiomyopathy as compared to restrictive pericarditis, likely owing to the decrease in myocardial compliance associated with fibrous infiltrates [83].

7. Surgical treatment of constrictive pericarditis

In 1898, the French physician, Dr. Delorme, first proposed surgical intervention in the treatment of pericarditis [84]. However, another fifteen years would pass before

Dr. Ludwig Rehn would perform the first successful pericardiectomy as a treatment for constrictive pericarditis [85]. In the United States, the first successful surgical treatment for constrictive pericarditis was performed by Dr. Edward Delos Churchill at Massachusetts General Hospital in 1928 [86]. The surgery has evolved since then and continues to be a mainstay of treatment for pericardial disease. Today, pericardiectomy is the gold standard of treatment for constrictive pericarditis and considered the only curative, rather than palliative, option. For most patients, medical therapy is only effective in the treatment of acute pericarditis, where corticosteroids and anti-inflammatory medications have shown to produce acceptable outcomes.

7.1 Indications for surgery

When determining whether a patient is a good candidate for pericardiectomy in the treatment of constrictive pericarditis, numerous factors must be taken into consideration. This procedure, while curative, is not without notable risks to the patient. Research into prognostic indicators is ongoing, though current recommendations focus on preoperative state and the patient's medical history,

Pericardiectomy produces the most positive outcomes in the treatment of constrictive pericarditis when performed early in the disease course [87, 88]. Clinical judgment is used to determine which patients are best suited to undergo pericardiectomy. Patients who fall into NYHA heart failure Classes I and II may remain clinically stable for years and be placed at unnecessary risk through surgery [41]. However, a delicate balance must be struck, as patients with advanced pericardial disease in NYHA Class IV who have significant left ventricular dysfunction or advanced fibrosis and calcification tend to have high mortality rates [41]. Therefore, outcomes depend largely on individual patient factors and a thorough risk-benefit analysis should be employed.

7.2 Midline sternotomy approach

The surgeon must not only determine whether the patient is a good candidate for pericardiectomy, but also which surgical technique is most appropriate given the patient's specific condition.

Approaching the pericardium through a median sternotomy is the most common technique used in the decortication procedure. This access provides the broadest view of the heart and its related structures, as well as the lungs and, crucially, the phrenic nerves.

The initial opening of the pericardium after a midline sternotomy may be easiest at the lower portion of the right ventricle, over the epicardial fat pad by the diaphragm. This provides the safest avenue of identifying the appropriate dissection planes, as the likelihood of damaging underlying structures is low. Dissection continues as the surgeon identifies the dissection plane that will separate the epicardium from its parietal pericardial adhesions, taking special care to avoid damaging the coronary vessels. It is also important to consider which portion of the heart will be decorticated first. Traditionally, the left ventricle is free first as, this helps to prevent pulmonary edema that may otherwise occur if the right ventricle were freed first. This particular approach can be quite challenging, though, and some surgeons elect to begin with the right ventricle and relieve the anterior plane first.

Avoiding damage to the underlying cardiac structures is of paramount importance when performing a pericardiectomy. As such, the surgeon must be cognizant of the dissection plane at all times. This can be particularly challenging in areas of especially thickened adhesions. In such instances, it may be necessary to dissect around a focal adhesion and perform a waffle procedure to minimize the risk of inadvertent damage to underlying myocardium. A waffle procedure involves making multiple longitudinal and transverse incisions in the thickened area of pericardium to create a more distensible surface.

As the surgical treatment for constrictive pericarditis has evolved and outcomes have been analyzed, the preferred techniques for removal of the pericardium have also changed. Historically, a partial, or anterior, pericardiectomy was performed. Following decortication of the mid-anterior portion of the pericardium, dissection proceeds laterally toward the phrenic nerves, carefully separating the planes of tissue and ending approximately 1 cm anterior to the nerves. Immediate hemodynamic improvement is observed upon removal of the diseased pericardium from the ventricles. The surgeon then turns their attention to the atria and all stiff pericardial tissue is resected. At completion, only the anterior section of the pericardium is removed, leaving the posterior surfaces adhered. While this approach is thought to be considerably less challenging and, therefore, safer than the alternative total pericardiectomy, it leaves intact any posterior adhesions and does not provide full resolution of the constriction. It also leaves an opportunity for further adhesions to form on the posterior surface of the heart and lead to progressively increased constriction and worsened hemodynamics. As will be discussed in more depth in the "Outcomes" section, patients who undergo partial pericardiectomy tend to experience sub-optimal outcomes and increased risk of complications [5, 8, 9].

Today, the more accepted approach is the total, or radical, pericardiectomy. Most modern studies report improved outcomes with total pericardiectomy. Improved hemodynamics, as measured by right ventricular pressures and reduced instances of tricuspid regurgitation, have been noted with complete pericardial removal as compared with the partial removal procedure [9]. Lower long term mortality rates have also been reported in total versus partial pericardiectomy [9]. Despite the more favorable outcomes of total pericardiectomy, some patients may be more suited to the partial approach. This includes those with advanced pericardial disease, poor cardiac function, or those at risk of acute heart failure following surgery [41].

This procedure begins at the right atrium, where the appropriate dissection plane is identified, and the right atrium is freed from its pericardial adhesions. This dissection continues to the level of the pulmonary veins and inferior vena cava. It is at this point that the right phrenic nerve is delicately removed as a fat pedicle, and the pericardium can be resected from around the entirety of the inferior vena cava. The surgeon then turns their attention to the left side of the heart, dissecting over the left atrium to the diaphragmatic surface of the heart, again taking special care around the coronary arteries and particularly dense adhesions. The left phrenic nerve is detached and protected as a fat pedicle. The dissection continues, detaching the pericardium from the diaphragm, pulmonary ligaments, posterior mediastinum, and major blood vessels until it can be extracted in its entirety.

Once all visible pericardial adhesions have been relieved, thoracic drains are inserted, the patient is monitored for hemodynamic stability, and echocardiography confirms appropriate cardiac blood flow.

7.3 Anterolateral thoracotomy

An alternative approach that is favored in some instances is the anterolateral thoracotomy. It provides for sufficient visualization of the lateral and diaphragmatic surfaces of the left ventricle without the need for excessive manipulation of the heart required of the midsternal approach. This approach is particularly beneficial for patients whose adhesions are primarily focused on the left side of the heart. It is less useful when the right side of the heart is involved as the field of view is very limited in that area.

The process of an anterolateral approach to pericardiectomy involves opening of the chest wall through the fourth or fifth intercostal space. If an expanded view is needed, the incision can be extended to the right side of the chest.

Once the thoracic cavity has been accessed, the left lung is displaced posteriorly, revealing the left side of the heart and left phrenic nerve. The pericardium is dissected anteriorly and posteriorly to the left phrenic nerve to a depth sufficient to identify the desired plane. Once the plane between the epicardium and parietal pericardium is localized, the pericardium is dissected away, beginning at the left ventricle, and proceeding over to the right ventricle. Finally, the adhesions overlying the pulmonary artery and aorta are removed, freeing the heart.

As previously stated, this approach does not allow for easy access to the right side of the heart. If pericardial adhesions extend to this area, it may be necessary to extend the thoracotomy to the right side of the chest. Then, a similar approach to that used on the left side can be taken to resolve any constrictions.

7.4 Cardiopulmonary bypass

Cardiopulmonary bypass in the surgical treatment of constrictive is not commonly utilized unless additional procedures are to be performed concomitantly and require it. More often, patients undergo the pericardiectomy with the femoral vessels prepared in case emergency bypass, but not as a standard part of the procedure. Having cardiopulmonary bypass at the ready can be useful in cases of extreme blood loss, large calcifications, or accidental damage to the heart during surgery [10].

Some research indicates that the use of cardiopulmonary bypass during a pericardiectomy procedure is an independent predictor of post-procedure complications [89]. It should be noted, though that because the use of cardiopulmonary bypass has traditionally been reserved for more hemodynamically unstable or higher-risk patients, it may not actually be a causative factor in negative outcomes but rather a marker for those already predisposed to such results [8]. Therefore, it seems to largely depend on surgeon preference whether a patient should undergo bypass during pericardial surgery.

8. Post-surgical prognoses

Post-pericardiectomy outcomes have been the subject of much study in recent years. Common avenues of research investigate the relationship between the etiology of constrictive pericarditis and surgical outcomes. As mentioned previously, the most common underlying causes of constrictive pericarditis include tuberculosis infection, previous cardiac surgery, mediastinal radiation, and idiopathic means [2–5, 10–15, 27, 30]. It appears that, despite the common resultant pathophysiology, unique causative etiologies are associated with variable long-term prognoses. One study reported that patients presenting with constrictive disease arising from tuberculosis infection and idiopathic sources tend to experience longer event-free survival than those having previously undergone cardiac surgery [90]. A second center found that the 5-year survival rate of patients treated for constrictive pericarditis arising from idiopathic causes stood at 79.8%, while those treated post-cardiac surgery or following mediastinal radiation demonstrated rates of 55.9% and 11.0%, respectively [13]. Previous mediastinal radiation, in particular, seems to be implicated with relative frequency in poor post-pericardiectomy outcomes [9].

Underlying etiology is not the only prognostic factor of post-surgical outcomes for constrictive pericarditis. Preexisting illness also seems to be significant contributor to patient prognosis. A retrospective study of patients at the Asian Medical Center found that diabetes mellitus represented an independent risk factor for post-procedure mortality, as did high early diastolic mitral inflow [91]. They also report that the patients who died following pericardiectomy had higher levels of aspartate aminotransferase, smaller left ventricular end-systolic dimension index, and higher early diastolic mitral inflow velocity prior to surgery compared with the patients who survived [91]. Other pre-surgery hemodynamic and structural parameters including reduced left ventricular ejection fraction, right ventricular dilation, central venous pressure, myocardial atrophy or fibrosis, and tricuspid regurgitation also appear to contribute to poor outcomes [41]. Perhaps unsurprisingly, advanced heart failure symptoms (NYHA III-IV) and arrhythmias are also associated with poor outcomes [41]. Likewise, advanced age and patients with end-stage renal disease, coronary artery disease, chronic obstructive pulmonary disease, sepsis, and other severe comorbidities also appear to experience poorer outcomes than other pericardiectomy patients [41, 92, 93].

9. Conclusions

While constrictive pericarditis represents a relatively rare disease process, it provides several diagnostic and treatment challenges. Constriction of the heart within the pericardium negatively impacts ventricular filling, leading to poor hemodynamics which, over time, can result in heart failure. Early diagnosis and management are key to improving patient prognoses and minimizing complications. Diagnosis of this condition requires a high degree of suspicion from the treating physician and a thorough exam. Imaging modalities, including computed tomography and cardiac magnetic resonance imaging, help to differentiate constrictive pericarditis from other conditions that may present with similar exam findings. Constrictive pericarditis responds poorly to medical management and typically requires surgical decortication of the fibrous adhesions holding the pericardium to the heart. The evolution of this procedure from the partial removal of the pericardium to the radical pericardiectomy has led to improved patient outcomes.

Conflict of interest

The authors declare no conflict of interest.

Author details

Juliana Cobb[1] and Siddharth Pahwa[2*]

1 University of Louisville, Louisville, Kentucky, United States

2 Department of Cardiovascular and Thoracic Surgery, University of Louisville, Louisville, Kentucky, United States

*Address all correspondence to: siddharth.pahwa@uoflhealth.org

IntechOpen

© 2023 The Author(s). Licensee IntechOpen. This chapter is distributed under the terms of the Creative Commons Attribution License (http://creativecommons.org/licenses/by/3.0), which permits unrestricted use, distribution, and reproduction in any medium, provided the original work is properly cited.

References

[1] Syed F, Schaff H, Oh J. Constrictive pericarditis—A curable diastolic heart failure. Nature Reviews Cardiology. 2014;**11**:530-544. DOI: 10.1038/nrcardio.2014.100

[2] Ling LH, Oh JK, Schaff HV, Danielson GK, Mahoney DW, Seward JB, et al. Constrictive pericarditis in the modern era: Evolving clinical spectrum and impact on outcome after pericardiectomy. Circulation. 1999;**100**(13):1380-1386. DOI: 10.1161/01.cir.100.13.1380

[3] Mayosi BM, Burgess LJ, Doubell AF. Tuberculous pericarditis. Circulation. 2005;**112**(23):3608-3616. DOI: 10.1161/CIRCULATIONAHA.105.543066

[4] Sagrista-Sauleda J, Permanyer-Miralda G, Soler-Soler J. Tuberculous pericarditis: Ten-year experience with a prospective protocol for diagnosis and treatment. Journal of the American College of Cardiology. 1988;**11**:724-728. DOI: 10.1016/0735-1097(88)90203-3

[5] Szabó G, Schmack B, Bulut C, Soós P, Weymann A, Stadtfeld S, et al. Constrictive pericarditis: Risks, aetiologies and outcomes after total pericardiectomy: 24 years of experience. European Journal of Cardio-Thoracic Surgery. 2013;**44**(6):1023-1028. DOI: 10.1093/ejcts/ezt138

[6] Muchtar E, Blauwet LA, Gertz MA. Restrictive cardiomyopathy—Genetics, pathogenesis, clinical manifestations, diagnosis, and therapy. Circulation Research. 2017;**121**(7):819-837. DOI: 10.1161

[7] Adler Y, Charron P, Imazio M, Badano L, Barón-Esquivias G, Bogaert J, et al. 2015 ESC guidelines for the diagnosis and management of pericardial diseases. European Heart Journal. 2015;**36**(42):2921-2964. DOI: 10.1093

[8] Unai S, Johnston DR. Radical pericardiectomy for pericardial diseases. Current Cardiology Reports. 2019;**21**(6). DOI: 10.1007/s11886-019-1092-1

[9] Choi MS, Jeong DS, Oh JK, Chang S, Park S, Suryeun C. Long-term results of radical pericardiectomy for constrictive pericarditis in Korean population. Journal of Cardiothoracic Surgery. 2019;**14**(32). DOI: 10.1186/s13019-019-0845-7

[10] Depboylu BC, Mootoosamy P, Vistarini N, Testuz A, El-Hamamsy I, Cikirikcioglu M. Surgical treatment of constrictive pericarditis. Texas Heart Institute Journal. 2017;**44**(2):101-106. DOI: 10.14503/THIJ-16-5772

[11] Cameron J, Oesterle SN, Baldwin JC, Hancock EW. The etiologic spectrum of constrictive pericarditis. American Heart Journal. 1987;**113**(2,1):354-360. DOI: 10.1016/0002-8703(87)90278-x

[12] Porta-Sánchez A, Sagristà-Sauleda J, Ferreira-González I, Torrents-Fernández A, Roca-Luque I, García-DoradoD.Constrictivepericarditis: Etiologic spectrum, patterns of clinical presentation, prognostic factors, and long-term follow-up. Revista Española de Cardiología. 2015;**68**(12):1092-1100. DOI: 10.1016/j.rec.2014.12.018

[13] George TJ, Arnaoutakis GJ, Beaty CA, Kilic A, Baumgartner WA, Conte JV. Contemporary etiologies, risk factors, and outcomes after pericardiectomy. The Annals of Thoracic Surgery. 2012;**94**(2):445-451. DOI: 10.1016/j.athoracsur.2012.03.079

[14] Vistarini N, Chen C, Mazine A, Bouchard D, Hebert Y, Carrier M, et al. Pericardiectomy for constrictive pericarditis: 20 years of experience at the Montreal Heart Institute. Annals of Thoracic Surgery. 2015;**100**(1):107-113. DOI: 10.1016/j.athoracsur.2015.02.054

[15] Imazio M, Brucato A, Derosa FG, Lestuzzi C, Bombana E, Scipione F, et al. Aetiological diagnosis in acute and recurrent pericarditis: When and how. Journal of Cardiovascular Medicine (Hagerstown). 2009;**10**(3):217-230. DOI: 10.2459/JCM.0b013e328322f9b1

[16] Miller H, Uricchio JF, Phillips RW. Acute pericarditis associated with infectious mononucleosis. New England Journal of Medicine. 1953;**249**:136-140. DOI: 10.1056/NEJM195307232490403

[17] Campbell PT, Li JS, Wall TC, O'Connor CM, Van Trigt P, Kenney RT, et al. Cytomegalovirus pericarditis: A case series and review of the literature. American Journal of Medical Science. 1995;**309**:229-234. DOI: 10.1097/00000441-199504000-00009

[18] Spoto S, Valeriani E, Locorriere L, Anguissola GB, Pantano AL, Terracciani F, et al. Influenza B virus infection complicated by life-threatening pericarditis: A unique case-report and literature review. BMC Infectious Disease. 2019;**19**(1):40. DOI: 10.1186/s12879-018-3606-7

[19] Rerkpattanapipat P, Wongpraparut N, Jacobs LE, Kotler MN. Cardiac manifestations of acquired immunodeficiency syndrome. Archives of Internal Medicine. 2000;**160**(5):602-608. DOI: 10.1001/archinte.160.5.602

[20] Lind A, Reinsch N, Neuhaus K, Esser S, Brockmeyer NH, Potthoff A, et al. Pericardial effusion of HIV-infected patients—Results of a prospective multicenter cohort study in the era of antiretroviral therapy. European Journal of Medical Research. 2011;**16**(11):480-483. DOI: 10.1186/2047-783x-16-11-480

[21] Heidenreich PA, Eisenberg MJ, Kee LL, Somelofski CA, Hollander H, Schiller NB, et al. Pericardial effusion in AIDS. Circulation. 1995;**92**:3229-3234. DOI: 10.1161/01.cir.92.11.3229

[22] Akpek M, Yarlioglueş M, Durmaz S, Kaya MG. İmmün sistemi normal genç bir hastada Epstein-Barr virüsü ile ilişkili perikart tamponadı [Pericardial tamponade associated with Epstein-Barr virus in an immunocompetent young patient]. Türk Kardiyoloji Derneği Arşivi. 2011;**39**(5):407-409. Turkish. DOI: 10.5543/tkda.2011.01312

[23] Lentini S, Klingel K, Skowasch D, Kandolf R, Bauriedel G. Epstein-Barr Virus assoziierte Perikarditis [Epstein-Barr virus-associated pericarditis]. Deutsche Medizinische Wochenschrift. 2001;**126**(38):1043-1046. German. DOI: 10.1055/s-2001-17307

[24] Zafrir B, Aviv A, Reichman N, Flatau E. Epstein-Barr virus-associated pericarditis and pericardial effusion: Case report and diagnostic aspects. European Journal of Internal Medicine. 2005;**16**(7):528-530. DOI: 10.1016/j.ejim.2005.09.006

[25] Hutter T, Springe D, Ebnöther L, Delgado M. Relevant pericardial effusion caused by cytomegalovirus infection in an immunocompetent patient: A case report. Journal of Medical Case Reports. 2018;**12**(1):14. DOI: 10.1186/s13256-017-1542-6

[26] Fernández-Ruiz M, Muñoz-Codoceo C, López-Medrano F, Faré-García R, Carbonell-Porras A, Garfia-Castillo C, et al. Cytomegalovirus myopericarditis and hepatitis

in an immunocompetent adult: Successful treatment with oral valganciclovir. Internal Medicine. 2008;**47**(22):1963-1966. DOI: 10.2169/internalmedicine.47.1480

[27] Tse G, Ali A, Alpendurada F, Prasad S, Raphael CE, Vassiliou V. Tuberculous constrictive pericarditis. Research in Cardiovascular Medicine. 2015;**4**(4):e29614. DOI: 10.5812/cardiovascmed.29614

[28] Petcu CP, Dilof R, Bătăiosu C, Petcu PD. Purulent pericardial effusions with pericardial tamponade—Diagnosis and treatment issues. Current Health Sciences Journal. 2013;**39**(1):53-56

[29] Oladele RO, Ayanlowo OO, Richardson MD, Denning DW. Histoplasmosis in Africa: An emerging or a neglected disease? PLoS Neglected Tropical Diseases. 2018;**12**(1):e0006046. DOI: 10.1371/journal.pntd.0006046

[30] Moreyra AE, Cosgrove NM, Zinonos S, Yang Y, Cabrera J, Pepe RJ, et al. Constrictive pericarditis after open heart surgery: A 20-year case controlled study. International Journal of Cardiology. 2021;**329**:63-66. DOI: 10.1016/j.ijcard.2020.12.090

[31] Pahwa S, Crestanello J, Miranda W, Bernabei A, Polycarpou A, Schaff H, et al. Outcomes of pericardiectomy for constrictive pericarditis following mediastinal irradiation. Journal of Cardiac Surgery. 2021;**36**(12):4636-4642. DOI: 10.1111/jocs.15996

[32] Khandaker MH, Espinosa RE, Nishimura RA, Sinak LJ, Hayes SN, Melduni RM, et al. Pericardial disease: Diagnosis and management. Mayo Clinic Proceedings. 2010;**85**(6):572-593. DOI: 10.4065/mcp.2010.0046

[33] Sunder SK, Shah A. Constrictive pericarditis in procainamide-induced lupus erythematosus syndrome. American Journal of Cardiology. 1975;**36**(7):960-962. DOI: 10.1016/0002-9149(75)90089-2

[34] McMechan SR, McClements BM, McKeown PP, Webb SW, Adgey AA. Systemic lupus erythematosus presenting as effuso-constrictive pericarditis. Postgraduate Medical Journal. 1995;**71**(840):627-629. DOI: 10.1136/pgmj.71.840.627

[35] Ho V, O'Sullivan J, Collins W, Ozdalga E, Bell CF, Shah ND, et al. Constrictive pericarditis revealing rare case of ALH amyloidosis with underlying lymphoplasmacytic lymphoma (Waldenstrom Macroglobulinemia). Journal of the American College of Cardiology Case Reports. 2022;**4**(5):271-275. DOI: 10.1016/j.jaccas.2022.01.007

[36] Singh V, Fishman JE, Alfonso CE. Primary systemic amyloidosis presenting as constrictive pericarditis. Cardiology. 2011;**118**(4):251-255. DOI: 10.1159/000329062

[37] Meaney E, Shabetai R, Bhargava V, Shearer M, Weidner C, Mangiardi LM, et al. Cardiac amyloidosis, contrictive pericarditis and restrictive cardiomyopathy. American Journal of Cardiology. 1976;**38**(5):547-556. DOI: 10.1016/s0002-9149(76)80001-x

[38] Valentin R, Keeley EC, Ataya A, Gomez-Manjarres D, Petersen J, Arnaoutakis GJ, et al. Breaking hearts and taking names: A case of sarcoidosis related effusive-constrictive pericarditis. Respiratory Medicine. 2020;**163**:105879. DOI: 10.1016/j.rmed.2020.105879

[39] Darda S, Zughaib ME, Alexander PB, Machado CE, David SW, Saba S. Cardiac sarcoidosis presenting as constrictive pericarditis. Texas Heart Institute

Journal. 2014;**41**(3):319-323. DOI: 10.14503/THIJ-13-3208

[40] Rehman KA, Betancor J, Xu B, Kumar A, Rivas CG, Sato K, et al. Uremic pericarditis, pericardial effusion, and constrictive pericarditis in end-stage renal disease: Insights and pathophysiology. Clinical Cardiology. 2017;**40**(10):839-846. DOI: 10.1002/clc.22770

[41] Matshela MR. Constrictive pericarditis: Prevention and treatment. European Society of Cardiology e-Journal of Cardiology Practice. 2017;**15**(24)

[42] Jaworska-Wilczynska M, Abramczuk E, Hryniewiecki T. Postcardiac injury syndrome. Medical Science Monitor. 2011;**17**(11):CQ13-CQ14. DOI: 10.12659/msm.882029

[43] Wada A, Craft J, Mazzaferri EL. Purulent pericarditis leading to constriction. Cardiology Research. 2014;**5**(6):188-190. DOI: 10.14740/cr356w

[44] Mehta A, Mehta M, Jain AC. Constrictive pericarditis. Clinical Cardiology. 1999;**22**(5):334-344. DOI: 10.1002/clc.4960220509

[45] Yun S, Vincelette ND, Mansour I, Hariri D, Motamed S. Late onset ipilimumab-induced pericarditis and pericardial effusion: A rare but life threatening complication. Case Reports in Oncology Medicine. 2015;**2015**:794842. DOI: 10.1155/2015/794842

[46] Moriyama S, Fukata M, Tatsumoto R, Kono M. Refractory constrictive pericarditis caused by an immune checkpoint inhibitor properly managed with infliximab: A case report. European Heart Journal Case Reports. 2021;**5**(1):ytab002. DOI: 10.1093/ehjcr/ytab002

[47] Saade A, Mansuet-Lupo A, Arrondeau J, Thibault C, Mirabel M, Goldwasser F, et al. Pericardial effusion under nivolumab: Case-reports and review of the literature. Journal for Immunotherapy of Cancer. 2019;**7**:266. DOI: 10.1186/s40425-019-0760-4

[48] Sakai T, Sasada S, Jyo C, Ishioka K, Takahashi S, Nakamura M. Acute myocarditis and pericarditis after nivolumab treatment in patients with non-small cell lung cancer. Annals of Oncology. 2017;**28**:IX90. DOI: 10.1093/annonc/mdx697.072

[49] Chiabrando JG, Bonaventura A, Vecchié A, Wohlford GF, Mauro AG, Jordan JH, et al. Management of acute and recurrent pericarditis: JACC state-of-the-art review. Journal of the American College of Cardiology. 2020;**75**(1):76-92. DOI: 10.1016/j.jacc.2019.11.021

[50] Kytö V, Sipilä J, Rautava P. Clinical profile and influences on outcomes in patients hospitalized for acute pericarditis. Circulation. 2014;**130**(18):1601-1606. DOI: 10.1161/CIRCULATIONAHA.114.010376

[51] Kyriakakis C, Herbst P, Doubell A. Constrictive pericarditis-prevalence, causes and clinical presentation. European Society of Cardiology e-Journal of Cardiology Practice. 2017;**15**(22)

[52] Chowdury UK, Seth S, Reddy SM. Pericardiectomy for chronic constrictive pericarditis via left anterolateral thoracotomy. Operative Techniques in Thoracic and Cardiovascular Surgery. 2008;**13**(1):14-25. DOI: 10.1053

[53] Geske JB, Reddy YNV. Pathophysiology and Diagnosis of

Constrictive Pericarditis [Internet]. 2017. Available from: https://www.acc.org/latest-in-cardiology/articles/2017/03/13/15/10/pathophysiology-and-diagnosis-of-constrictive-pericarditis. [Accessed: November 20, 2022]

[54] El-Sherif A, El-Said G. Jugular, hepatic, and praecordial pulsations in constrictive pericarditis. British Heart Journal. 1971;**33**(2):305-312. DOI: 10.1136/hrt.33.2.305

[55] Murashita T, Hartzell V, Schaff HV, Richard C, Daly RC, Oh JK, et al. Experience with pericardiectomy for constrictive pericarditis over eight decades. Annals of Thoracic Surgery. 2017;**104**(3):742-750. DOI: 10.1016/j.athoracsur.2017.05.063

[56] Oh JK, Hatle LK, Seward JB, Danielson GK, Schaff HV, Reeder GS, et al. Diagnostic role of Doppler echocardiography in constrictive pericarditis. Journal of the American College of Cardiology. 1994;**23**(1):154-162. DOI: 10.1016/0735-1097(94)90514-2

[57] Hoit BD. Imaging the pericardium. Cardiology Clinics. 1990;**8**(4):587-600

[58] D'Cruz IA, Dick A, Gross CM, Hand CR, Lalmalani GG. Abnormal left ventricular-left atrial posterior wall contour: A new two-dimensional echocardiographic sign in constrictive pericarditis. American Heart Journal. 1989;**118**(1):128-132. DOI: 10.1016/0002-8703(89)90082-3

[59] Troughton RW, Asher CR, Klein AL. Pericarditis. Lancet. 2004;**363**(9410):717-727. DOI: 10.1016/S0140-6736(04)15648-1

[60] Talreja DR, Edwards WD, Danielson GK, Schaff HV, Tajik AJ, Tazelaar HD, et al. Constrictive pericarditis in 26 patients with histologically normal pericardial thickness. Circulation. 2003;**108**(15):1852-1857. DOI: 10.1161/01.CIR.0000087606.18453.FD

[61] Engel PJ, Fowler NO, Tei CW, Shah PM, Driedger HJ, Shabetai R, et al. M-mode echocardiography in constrictive pericarditis. Journal of the American College of Cardiology. 1985;**6**(2):471-474. DOI: 10.1016/s0735-1097(85)80188-1

[62] Boonyaratavej S, Oh JK, Tajik AJ, Appleton CP, Seward JB. Comparison of mitral inflow and superior vena cava Doppler velocities in chronic obstructive pulmonary disease and constrictive pericarditis. Journal of the American College of Cardiology. 1998;**32**(7):2043-2048. DOI: 10.1016/s0735-1097(98)00472-0

[63] Schnittger I, Bowden RE, Abrams J, Popp RL. Echocardiography: Pericardial thickening and constrictive pericarditis. American Journal of Cardiology. 1978;**42**(3):388-395. DOI: 10.1016/0002-9149(78)90933-5

[64] Agatston AS, Rao A, Price RJ, Kinney EL. Diagnosis of constrictive pericarditis by pulsed Doppler echocardiography. American Journal of Cardiology. 1984;**54**(7):929-930. DOI: 10.1016/s0002-9149(84)80241-6

[65] Klein AL, Cohen GI, Pietrolungo JF, White RD, Bailey A, Pearce GL, et al. Differentiation of constrictive pericarditis from restrictive cardiomyopathy by Doppler transesophageal echocardiographic measurements of respiratory variations in pulmonary venous flow. Journal of the American College of Cardiology. 1993;**22**(7):1935-1943. DOI: 10.1016/0735-1097(93)90782-v

[66] Wang ZJ, Reddy GP, Gotway MB, Yeh BM, Hetts SW, Higgins CB. CT and MR imaging of pericardial disease. RadioGraphics. 2003;**23**(suppl. 1):S167-S180. DOI: 10.1148/rg.23si035504

[67] Ariyarajah V, Jassal DS, Kirkpatrick I, Kwong RY. The utility of cardiovascular magnetic resonance in constrictive pericardial disease. Cardiology Reviews. 2009;**17**(2):77-82. DOI: 10.1097/CRD.0b013e318197e950

[68] Cosyns B, Plein S, Nihoyanopoulos P, Smiseth O, Achenbach S, Andrade MJ, et al. On behalf of the European Association of Cardiovascular Imaging (EACVI) and European Society of Cardiology Working Group (ESC WG) on Myocardial and Pericardial diseases, European Association of Cardiovascular Imaging (EACVI) position paper: Multimodality imaging in pericardial disease. European Heart Journal - Cardiovascular Imaging. 2015;**16**(1):12-31. DOI: 10.1093/ehjci/jeu128

[69] Velthuis S, Laufer E, Hofstra L, Minkens MHM. An armored heart in constrictive pericarditis. Journal of the American College of Cardioogyl. 2009;**53**(11):972. DOI: 10.1016/j.jacc.2008.11.045

[70] Chesler E, Mitha AS, Matisonn RE. The ECG of constrictive pericarditis—Pattern resembling right ventricular hypertrophy. American Heart Journal. 1976;**91**(4):420-424. DOI: 10.1016/s0002-8703(76)80321-3

[71] Rezaian GR, Poor-Moghaddas M, Kojuri J, Rezaian S, Liaghat L, Zare N. Atrial fibrillation in patients with constrictive pericarditis: The significance of pericardial calcification. Annals of Noninvasive Electrocardiology. 2009;**14**(3):258-261. DOI: 10.1111/j.1542-474X.2009.00307.x

[72] Doshi S, Ramakrishnan S, Gupta SK. Invasive hemodynamics of constrictive pericarditis. Indian Heart Journal. 2015;**67**(2):175-182. DOI: 10.1016

[73] Hurrell DG, Nishimura RA, Higano ST, Appleton CP, Danielson GK, Holmes DR Jr, et al. Value of dynamic respiratory changes in left and right ventricular pressures for the diagnosis of constrictive pericarditis. Circulation. 1996;**93**(11):2007-2013. DOI: 10.1161/01.cir.93.11.2007

[74] Bertog SC, Thambidorai SK, Parakh K, Schoenhagen P, Ozduran V, Houghtaling PL, et al. Constrictive pericarditis: Etiology and cause-specific survival after pericardiectomy. Journal of the American College of Cardiology. 2004;**43**(8):1445-1452. DOI: 10.1016/j.jacc.2003.11.048

[75] Mutyaba AK, Balkaran S, Cloete R, du Plessis N, Badri M, Brink J, et al. Constrictive pericarditis requiring pericardiectomy at Groote Schuur Hospital, Cape Town, South Africa: Causes and perioperative outcomes in the HIV era (1990-2012). The Journal of Thoracic and Cardiovascular Surgery. 2014;**148**(6):3058-3065. DOI: 10.1016/j.jtcvs.2014.07.065

[76] Cyrille NB, Goldsmith J, Alvarez J, Maurer MS. Prevalence and prognostic significance of low QRS voltage among the three main types of cardiac amyloidosis. American Journal Cardiology. 2014;**114**(7):1089-1093. DOI: 10.1016/j.amjcard.2014.07.026

[77] Leya FS, Arab D, Joyal D, Shioura KM, Lewis BE, Steen LH, et al. The efficacy of brain natriuretic peptide levels in differentiating constrictive pericarditis from restrictive cardiomyopathy. Journal of the American College of Cardiology. 2005;**45**(11):1900-2000. DOI: 10.1016/j.jacc.2005.03.050

[78] Babuin L, Alegria JR, Oh JK, Nishimura RA, Jaffe AS. Brain natriuretic peptide levels in constrictive pericarditis and restrictive cardiomyopathy. Journal of the American College of Cardiology. 2006;**47**(7):1489-1491. DOI: 10.1016/j.jacc.2006.01.007

[79] Sengupta PP, Krishnamoorthy VK, Abhayaratna WP, Korinek J, Belohlavek M, Sundt TM 3rd, et al. Comparison of usefulness of tissue Doppler imaging versus brain natriuretic peptide for differentiation of constrictive pericardial disease from restrictive cardiomyopathy. American Journal of Cardiology. 2008;**102**(3):357-362. DOI: 10.1016/j.amjcard.2008.03.068

[80] Yang CC, Tsai CS, Tsai YT, Lin CY, Chen JL, Hsu PS. Restrictive cardiomyopathy caused by diffuse calcification of the left ventricle after 20 years of haemodialysis. Cardiovascular Journal of Africa. 2022;**33**(2):95-97. DOI: 10.5830/CVJA-2021-031

[81] Masui T, Finck S, Higgins CB. Constrictive pericarditis and restrictive cardiomyopathy: Evaluation with MR imaging. Radiology. 1992;**182**(2):369-373. DOI: 10.1148/radiology.182.2.1732952

[82] Rajagopalan N, Garcia MJ, Rodriguez L, Murray RD, Apperson-Hansen C, Stugaard M, et al. Comparison of new Doppler echocardiographic methods to differentiate constrictive pericardial heart disease and restrictive cardiomyopathy. American Journal of Cardiology. 2001;**87**(1):86-94. DOI: 10.1016/s0002-9149(00)01278-9

[83] Amaki M, Savino J, Ain DL, Sanz J, Pedrizzetti G, Kulkarni H, et al. Diagnostic concordance of echocardiography and cardiac magnetic resonance-based tissue tracking for differentiating constrictive pericarditis from restrictive cardiomyopathy. Circulation Cardiovascular Imaging. 2014;**7**(5):819-827. DOI: 10.1161/CIRCIMAGING.114.002103

[84] Delorme E. Sur un traitement chirurgical: De la symphyse cardopéricardique. Gaz Des Hôp. 1898;**71**:1150-1151

[85] Rehn L. Ueber pericardiale Verwachsungen. Medizinische Klinik. 1920;**16**:991

[86] Churchill ED. Decortication of the heart (Delorme) for adhesive pericarditis. Archivals of Surgery. 1929;**19**:1457

[87] Tiruvoipati R, Naik RD, Loubani M, Billa GN. Surgical approach for pericardiectomy: A comparative study between median sternotomy and left anterolateral thoracotomy. Interactive CardioVascular and Thoracic Surgery. 2003;**2**(3):322-326. DOI: 10.1016/S1569-9293(03)00074-4

[88] Srivastava AK, Ganjoo AK, Misra B, Chaterjee T, Kapoor A, Pandey CM. Subtotal pericardiectomy via sternotomy for constrictive pericarditis. Asian Cardiovascular and Thoracic Annals. 2000;**8**(2):134-136. DOI: 10.1177/021849230000800210

[89] Gatti G, Fiore A, Ternacle J, Porcari A, Fiorica I, Poletti A, et al. Pericardiectomy for constrictive pericarditis: A risk factor analysis for early and late failure. Heart and Vessels. 2019;**35**(1):92-103. DOI: 10.1007/s00380-019-01464-4

[90] Nishimura S, Izumi C, Amano M, Imamura S, Onishi N, Tamaki Y, et al. Long-term clinical outcomes and prognostic factors after pericardiectomy for constrictive pericarditis in a Japanese population. Circulation Journal. 2017;**81**:206-212. DOI: 10.1253/circj.CJ-16-0633